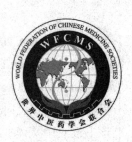

Guidance for Managing Ethical Issues in Infectious Disease Outbreaks

世界卫生组织授权
世界中医药学会联合会伦理审查委员会翻译

传染病暴发伦理问题管理指南

译　熊宁宁　王思成　刘海涛　伍　蓉　沈一峰
　　白　桦　徐春波　刘　强　申　丹
校　胡庆澧　邱仁宗

全国百佳图书出版单位
中国中医药出版社
·北京·

世界卫生组织于 2016 年发布，题为《传染病暴发伦理问题管理指南》

Guidance for Managing Ethical Issues in Infectious Disease Outbreaks

© World Health Organization (2016)

世界卫生组织已向世界中医药学会联合会伦理审查委员会授予中文版本的翻译和出版许可，
该书仅对中文译本的质量和真实性负责。中英文版本如有歧义，以英文本为准。

图书在版编目（CIP）数据

传染病暴发伦理问题管理指南 / 世界卫生组织授权；熊宁宁等译 . —北京：中国中医药出版社，2021.6
ISBN 978-7-5132-6135-7

Ⅰ . ①传… Ⅱ . ①世… ②熊… Ⅲ . ①传染病－卫生管理－医学伦理学－指南 Ⅳ . ① R184-62

中国版本图书馆 CIP 数据核字（2020）第 028425 号

中国中医药出版社出版

北京经济技术开发区科创十三街 31 号院二区 8 号楼
邮政编码 100176
传真 010-64405721
三河市同力彩印有限公司印刷
各地新华书店经销

开本 889×1194 1/16 印张 8 字数 226 千字
2021 年 6 月第 1 版 2021 年 6 月第 1 次印刷
书号 ISBN 978－7－5132－6135－7

定价 58.00 元
网址 www.cptcm.com

社 长 热 线 010-64405720
购 书 热 线 010-89535836
维 权 打 假 010-64405753

微信服务号 zgzyycbs
微商城网址 https://kdt.im/LIdUGr
官 方 微 博 http://e.weibo.com/cptcm
天猫旗舰店网址 https://zgzyycbs.tmall.com

如有印装质量问题请与本社出版部联系（010-64405510）

由世界卫生组织授权世界中医药学会联合会伦理审查委员会翻译并出版

目录

前　言

　　传染病暴发是一个充满不确定性的时期。随着事态的发展，往往有限的资源和能力进一步捉襟见肘，尽管决策的证据可能很少，却必须迅速作出公共卫生应对的决定。在这种情况下，公共卫生官员、政策制定者、资助者、研究人员、现场流行病学家、急救人员、国家伦理委员会、卫生保健工作人员和公共卫生从业人员需要一个道德指针来指导他们作出决策。生命伦理学将人置于问题的核心，强调这应当作为指导卫生体系的原则，并为作出选择尤其是危机中的选择提供了道德基础。

　　因此，我欢迎《传染病暴发伦理问题管理指南》的制定，这对于将伦理纳入针对传染病的流行和其他公共卫生紧急情况的全球综合警报和应对系统至关重要。该指南的出版还将支持和加强在这种情况下实施和采用的政策和计划。

　　研究是公共卫生应对措施中不可或缺的一个组成部分——不仅要了解当前的传染病的流行，而且要为未来的流行建立证据基础。传染病流行期间的研究范围包括流行病学、社会行为学、临床试验和毒性研究，所有这些都是至关重要的。我很高兴看到该指南在这个重要领域提供了建议，这不仅涉及未经证实的干预措施的研究和紧急使用，而且还涉及快速数据共享，请参见：http://www.who.int/ihr/procedures/ SPG_data_sharing.pdf?ua=1.

　　在传染病暴发期间，对沟通交流的重视与否可能使公共卫生所做的努力获得成功，或可能使之归于失败，世界卫生组织对此非常重视。本文件概述了应当作为指导从一线工作人员到政策制定者各个层面的沟通交流计划和实施的伦理原则。

　　该指南的制定，国际利益攸关方和专家组成的国际小组做了大量工作，其中包括负责地方、国家和国际各级应对管理的公共卫生从业人员，非政府组织代表，资助机构的主管，伦理委员会主席，研究实验室负责人，国家监管机构的代表，患者代表，以及公共卫生伦理学、生命伦理学、人权、人类学和流行病学方面的专家。我感谢他们的支持和投入。

Dr Marie–Paule Kieny

Assistant Director–General

Health Systems and Innovation

致 谢

这份指南是在全球卫生伦理学团队协调员 Abha Saxena 的总体指导下编写的，Andreas Reis 和 Maria Magdalena Guraiib 提供了支持。

世界卫生组织感谢 Carl Coleman 担任主要作者，他分析和综合了现有的指导文件，并将筹备会议和更广泛的同行审查过程中产生的意见纳入其中。

感谢对指南文件草稿提出意见的许多个人和组织，其中包括：Alice Desclaux, Institut de Recherche pour le Développement, France; Aminu Yakubu, Federal Ministry of Health, Nigeria; Annick Antierens, Médecins Sans Frontières, Belgium; Bagher Larijani, Endocrinology and Metabolism Research Center, Iran (Islamic Republic of); Brad Freeman, Washington University School of Medicine, USA; Catherine Hankins, Amsterdam Institute for Global Health and Development, Netherlands; Cheryl Macpherson, Bioethics Department, St. George's University School of Medicine, Grenada; Claude Vergès, Universidad de Panamá, Panama; Drue H Barrett, Nicole J Cohen, and Rita F Helfand, Centers for Disease Control and Prevention, USA; Dirceu Greco, Federal University of Minas Gerais, Brazil; Edward Foday, Ministry of Health and Sanitation, Sierra Leone; Emilie Alirol, Geneva University Hospitals, Switzerland; Heather Draper, University of Birmingham, United Kingdom; Kenneth Goodman, Miller School of Medicine, University of Miami, USA; Morenike Oluwatoyin Ukpong, Obafemi Awolowo University, Nigeria; Paul Bouvier, International Committee of the Red Cross, Switzerland; Ruth Macklin, Albert Einstein College of Medicine, USA; Voo Tech Chuan, Centre for Biomedical Ethics, National University of Singapore, Singapore.

我们还要感谢下列机构的建议、评论和指导：COST Action IS 1201: Disaster Bioethics (in particular Dónal O'Mathúna, Dublin City University, Ireland; the staff of the Nuffield Council on Bioethics, United Kingdom (in particular Hugh Whittall); Johns Hopkins Berman Institute of Bioethics, USA (in particular Nancy Kass and Jeffrey Kahn); the International Severe Acute Respiratory and Emerging Infection Consortium, United Kingdom and its members (in particular Alistair Nichol, Irish Critical Care–Clinical Research Core, University College Dublin, Ireland, and Raul Pardinaz-Solis, Centre for Tropical Medicine and Global Health, University of Oxford, United Kingdom); and the

Secretariat of the National Committee of Bioethics, King Abdulaziz City for Science and Technology, Kingdom of Saudi Arabia.

世界卫生组织感谢主席（Christiane Woopen，当时的德国伦理学理事会主席）与国家伦理／生命伦理学委员会全球峰会指导委员会成员的合作，他们于 2016 年 3 月在柏林举行的峰会上向 83 个国家伦理委员会的代表提交了该指南的较早草案。他们的评论和意见已纳入本文件。

该文件还受益于世界卫生组织生命伦理学全球网络合作中心对它的审阅。特别感谢该网络中心即将卸任的主席 Ronald Bayer 和公共卫生监测伦理学准则制定小组主席 Amy Fairchild（均来自美国哥伦比亚大学梅尔曼公共卫生学院），以及新任的该网络中心主席，澳大利亚莫纳什大学人类生命伦理学研究中心的 Michael Selgelid。这些人的总结性评价确保了指南文件与其他正在进行的研究计划是一致的。

许多在流行病暴发期间受到常规性挑战的一线工作人员和世界卫生组织工作人员，根据其个人经验提供了宝贵的帮助，使该文件的内容更加丰富。世界卫生组织研究伦理学委员会和公共卫生伦理学咨询小组提供了宝贵的意见，尤其是吸收了他们对埃博拉和寨卡病毒暴发期间进行的研究和公共卫生研究计划的审查意见。

世界卫生组织感谢加拿大多伦多大学的 Ross Upshur（伦理学工作组的第一任主席），以及后任的共同主席，加拿大麦克马斯特大学的 Lisa Schwartz 和塞内加尔达喀尔巴斯德研究所的 Aissatou Touré 的意见。两位共同主席花了无数小时与秘书处和首席撰稿人一起仔细审查收到的许多意见，并最后确定文件的形式。伦理学专家小组主席，瑞士无国界医生组织的 Philippe Calain，以及各个伦理学工作组成员，不断向世界卫生组织秘书处提出要求，要求其越过科学，关注受疫情影响的人群以及他们的文化和社会。

指南文件特别受益于世界卫生组织以下工作人员的审阅意见：Juliet Bedford, Carla Saenz Bresciani, Ian Clarke, Rudi J J M Coninx, Pierre Formenty, Gaya Manori Gamhewage, Theo Grace, Paul Gully, Brooke Ronald Johnson JR, Annette Kuesel, Anaïs Legand, Ahmed Mohamed Amin Mandil, Bernadette Murgue, Tim Nguyen, Asiya Ismail Odugleh-Kolev, Martin Matthew Okechukwu Ota, Bruce Jay Plotkin, Annie Portela, Marie-Pierre Preziosi, Manju Rani, Nigel Campbell Rollins, Cathy Roth, Manisha Shridhar, Rajesh Sreedharan, David Wood, and Yousef Elbes.

特别感谢负责伦理学工作组管理工作的 Vâniade la FuenteNúñez 和负责协调整个过程的 Michele Loi。全球卫生伦理学小组的前实习生 Patrick Hummel（英国圣安德鲁斯大学）和 Corinna Klingler（德国慕尼黑大学）需要特别提及，他们进行了有关妊娠和传染病的较大范围的调查，为这一领域的指南的制定提供了信息。

没有威康信托基金会的慷慨支持，这份指南是不可能完成的。我们也非常感谢以下合作伙伴的善意支持：3U 全球卫生伙伴关系；加拿大卫生研究所；都柏林城市大学；欧盟科学和技术合作项目；莫纳什大学；迈阿密大学米勒医学院生命伦理与卫生政策研究所。

绪　论

　　这份指南源于世界卫生组织（WHO）对 2014 年至 2016 年西非埃博拉疫情暴发引发的伦理问题的关注。WHO 全球卫生伦理小组对埃博拉病毒的应对始于 2014 年 8 月，当时根据《国际卫生条例（2005），IHR》[1]，埃博拉病毒疫情被宣布为"国际关注的突发公共卫生事件"。那次宣布促使成立了一个伦理学专家组以及之后的一个伦理学工作组，负责就传染病流行过程中出现的问题和关注点制定伦理指南。越来越明显的是，埃博拉引发的伦理问题反映了在全球性其他传染病暴发中出现的问题，包括严重急性呼吸道综合征（SARS）、流感大流行和多重耐药的结核病。然而，尽管 WHO 对其中一些传染病暴发颁发了伦理指南 [2,3,4,5]，但先前的指南仅针对分离的特定病原体。本指南的目的不再局限于特定传染病病原体，将重点放在对传染病暴发普遍适用的跨领域的伦理问题上。除了提出一般原则外，本指南还研究了如何使这些原则适用于不同的传染病流行情况和社会情况。

　　虽然传染病暴发中出现的许多伦理问题与其他公共卫生领域中出现的问题相同，但暴发的背景具有特殊的复杂性。传染病暴发期间需要紧急作出决定，而且通常是处在科学的不确定性、社会和机构混乱，以及恐惧和不信任的总体氛围的情况下。情况通常如此：受疫情暴发影响最严重的国家资源有限，法律和监管结构不完善，卫生系统缺乏应对危机局势的应变能力。经历自然灾害和武装冲突的国家尤其面临风险，因为这些情况同时增加了传染病暴发的风险，也同时减少了所需的资源和获得卫生保健的机会。此外，传染病暴发可能产生或加剧社会危机，从而削弱本已脆弱的卫生系统。在这样的情况下，不可能同时满足所有的紧急需要，迫使决策者权衡具有潜在冲突的伦理价值取向并确定优先顺序。时间的压力和资源的限制可能迫使行动缺乏充分的审议、包容和透明度，而这正是一个完善的符合伦理的决策过程所要求的。

　　本指南专门针对传染病暴发背景下出现的伦理问题，旨在补充现有的公共卫生伦理指南。因此，在阅读时应结合有关公共卫生监测、涉及人类参与者的研究以及解决脆弱群体需要等问题的更具普适性的指南。

　　提前建立决策系统和程序是确保在疫情暴发时作出伦理学上合适决策的最佳方式。鼓励各国、卫生保健机构、国际组织和其他参与传染病流行应对工作的机构在考虑到当地社会、文化和政治背景的情况下，制定切实可行的策略和方法，将本指南中的原则应用于其具体环境。WHO

致力于向各国提供技术援助，以支持这些努力。

相关伦理原则

伦理学涉及对"我们应有的生活方式，如我们的行动、意图和习惯行为"的判断[3]。伦理分析的过程包括识别相关的原则，将它们应用于特定的情况，并在无法满足所有原则的情况下，就如何权衡相互冲突的原则作出判断。本指南引用了各种伦理原则，并将其分为以下七个大类。这些分类仅仅是为了方便读者而提出的；其他分类方法也同样合理。

公正——在本文中，公正或公平包含两个不同的概念。第一个是分配公正，是指资源、机会和后果分配的公平。分配公正的关键要素包括一视同仁，避免歧视和剥削，对特别容易受到伤害或不公正的人保持敏感。公正的第二个方面是程序公正，指的是作出重要决定的公平程序。程序公正的要素包括正当程序（向有关人士发出通知，并有机会发表意见）、透明性（提供关于决策依据和他们借以作出决策的程序的清晰准确信息）、包容性/社区参与（确保所有利益攸关方能够参与决策）、问责（分配和执行决策的责任）以及监督（确保合适的监测和审查机制）。

有益——有益是指使他人受益而作出的行为，如努力减轻个人的疼痛和痛苦。在公共卫生方面，有益原则是社会有义务满足个人和社区的基本需要，特别是人道主义需要，如营养、住所、健康和安全的基础。

效用——效用原则是指只要行动能促进个人或社区的福祉，它就是正确的。努力实现效用最大化要求考虑相称性（平衡一项活动的潜在受益与伤害的风险）和效率（以可能最低的成本实现最大的受益）。

尊重人——"尊重人"一词是指以符合和承认我们共同人性、尊严和固有权利的方式对待个人。尊重人的核心是尊重自主性，这要求允许个人根据自己的价值观和偏好作出自己的选择。知情同意是落实这一概念的一种方式，即有行为能力的个人根据充分的相关信息授权采取行动的一个过程，而不受胁迫或不当引诱。如果个人缺乏决策能力，则可能需要由其他人负责保护其利益。尊重人还包括注意隐私和保密，以及社会、宗教、文化信仰和重要关系，包括家庭纽带。最后，在开展公共卫生和研究活动时，尊重人要求信息透明和讲真话。

自由——自由包括范围广泛的社会、宗教和政治自由，如行动自由、和平集会的自由以及言论自由。自由的许多方面作为基本人权受到保护。

互惠——互惠包括对人们所做的贡献进行"适当的和相称的回报"[6]。鼓励互惠的政策可能是促进公正原则的重要手段，因为它们可以纠正在传染病流行应对工作中受益和负担分配方面的不公平差异。

团结——团结是使群体、社区、国家或潜在的全球共同体联合在一起的社会关系[7]。团结原则为面对共同威胁采取集体行动提供辩护。本原则还支持尽量克服损害少数群体和受歧视群体福利的不平等。

实际应用

伦理原则的应用应当尽可能知晓可得到的证据。例如，在确定某一特定行动是否有效时，决策者应当以预期受益和伤害的任何可得的科学证据为指导。所提议的行动越具有侵入性，就越需要强有力的证据，证明所提议的行动有可能实现其预期目标。在没有具体证据的情况下，决定应尽可能基于理由充分的实质性意见，并知晓类似情况的证据。

在传染病暴发期间平衡相互冲突的原则时，各国必须尊重其根据国际人权协定承担的义务。《公民权利和政治权利国际公约》（"锡拉库萨原则"）[8]中"关于限制和减损条款的锡拉库萨原则"是一个广泛接受的框架，用于评估在紧急情况下限制某些基本人权的合适性。锡拉库萨原则规定，对人权的任何限制必须遵循法律和符合广大群众利益的正当目标来执行。此外，这些限制必须是绝对必要的，而且必须在采用其他侵入性程度较低的手段无法达到同一目的的情况下。最后，任何限制都必须以科学证据为基础，而不是以武断、不合理或歧视性的方式强加于人。出于务实和伦理的理由，保持人群对传染病流行应对工作的信任至关重要。只有政策制定者和应对工作者以可信任的方式行事，公平和一贯地应用程序原则，对基于最新相关信息的审查持开放态度，并在受影响社区的真正投入下一起行动，这种信任才有可能。此外，协调一致对于任何应对工作的成功都是必不可少的。全球社会的所有成员都需要同舟共济地采取行动，因为所有国家都容易受到传染病的威胁。

指南是如何制定的

许多人直接或间接地帮助制定本指南，首先是总干事于2014年8月11日召集的伦理学专家小组，以及2014年8月至10月在瑞士日内瓦召开的特设伦理学工作组会议，就西非埃博拉疫情期间未经测试的干预措施的使用提供指导。随后，2015年5月，一个专家组和利益攸关方在爱尔兰都柏林举行会议，审查关于传染病暴发的现有伦理声明，并制定创建更全面文件的方法。为协助这一进程，准备了关于与传染病暴发伦理考虑有关的所有现有指南文件的分析和综合（附件1）。与会者在反思以往疫情暴发的教训，特别是最近埃博拉疫情的经验时强调，需要针对不同的传染病流行、社会和经济背景提供指南。他们还讨论了全球卫生治理、社区参与、知识产生和优先事项设置等更广泛问题的重要性。最后，与会者强调，迫切需要提出具体的实施方法，帮助参与传染病流行应对工作的个人将伦理指南纳入实际决策。该小组于2015年11月在意大利普拉托再次举行会议，审议了指南的初稿，并听取了其他专家和利益攸关方的意见，包括最近埃博拉疫情的幸存者。这次会议之后，拟订了一份新的草案，并分发给国际同行审议。参加这些会议编写《准则》的专家名单载于附件2。

本指南由14条具体准则组成，每条准则都涉及传染病流行防控规划和应对的关键方面。每条准则都提出一系列问题，说明伦理问题的范围，然后进行更详细的讨论，阐明相关利益攸关方的权利和义务。希望这份指南可以对下列人员提供帮助：政策制定者、公共卫生专业人员、卫生保健工作人员、一线工作人员、研究人员、制药和医疗器械公司，以及公共和私营部门中涉及传染病暴发防控规划和应对行动的其他相关实体。

传染病暴发伦理问题管理指南

准 则

1. 政府和国际社会的义务

> **要解决的问题：**
> · 政府在预防和应对传染病暴发方面有哪些义务？
> · 为什么国家预防和应对传染病暴发的义务超越他们本国边界？
> · 各国在参与全球监测和防范工作中必须尽哪些义务？
> · 政府有哪些义务必须向有需要的国家提供财政、技术和科学援助？

政府可以通过改善社会和环境条件、确保卫生系统的良好运转和可及性，以及开展公共卫生监测和预防活动，在预防和应对传染病暴发方面发挥关键作用。这些行动可以大大减少具有流行潜力的疾病传播。此外，它们有助于确保在疫情发生时能够采取有效的公共卫生应对措施。各国政府负有伦理义务来确保长期系统地实施有效的传染病流行预防和应对行动。

各国不仅对其境内的个人负有义务，而且对更广泛的国际社会负有义务。正如联合国经济、社会和文化权利委员会所认可的那样，"鉴于某些疾病很容易跨越国家边界传播，国际社会对解决这一问题负有集体责任。在这方面，经济发达的国家尤其负有特殊责任并参与来帮助较贫穷的发展中国家"。[9]

这些义务反映了这样一个现实，即传染病暴发没有国界，一个国家的暴发可能使世界其他地区处于危险之中。

各国关注国际社会需要的义务并不只是在紧急情况下才产生。相反，这些义务要求持续关注改善导致传染病暴发的不健康的社会因素，包括贫困、有限的受教育机会、不完善的供水和环卫系统。

以下是各国政府和国际社会义务的关键要素：

• 确保国家公共卫生法律的充分性——如本指南后面讨论的那样，在传染病暴发期间可能需要的某些公共卫生干预措施（例如限制行动自由）有赖于政府行动有明确法律依据，以及合适的监督和审查体系。所有国家都应审查其公共卫生法，以确保赋予政府足够的权力，以有效应对传染病流行，同时向个人提供合适的人权保护。

• 参与全球监测和防范工作——所有国家必须履行《国际卫生条例》规定的责任，以诚实和透明的方式参与全球监测工作。这包括迅速通报可能构成国际关注的突发公共卫生事件，而不考虑通报可能带来的任何负面后果，如可能减少贸易或旅游。快速向国际社会提供通报的义务不仅源于《国际卫生条例》的文本，而且也源于团结和互惠的伦理原则。此外，各国应制定传染病暴发和其他潜在灾害的应对预案，并为实施这些计划相关的卫生保健机构提供指导。

- 提供财政、技术和科学援助——拥有向国外提供援助资源的国家应当支持全球传染病流行的防范和应对行动，包括对具有流行潜力的病原体的诊断、治疗和疫苗的研究和开发。对于受传染病暴发伤害风险最大的国家，这种支持应当是对这些国家建设地方公共卫生能力和加强初级卫生保健体系所作努力的补充。

2. 当地社区参与

要解决的问题：

- 为什么社区参与是传染病暴发的应对行动的一个关键组成部分？
- 以社区为中心的方式应对传染病暴发有何特点？
- 决策者应当如何处理他们在社区参与活动中获得的信息？
- 在传染病暴发的应对行动中，媒体的作用是什么？

传染病暴发应对行动的所有方面都应当得到受影响社区的早期和持续参与的支持。社区参与除了在伦理上很重要之外，对建立和维护信任以及维护社会秩序至关重要。

让社区充分参与传染病暴发的规划和应对行动，要求注意以下问题：

- 包容性——所有可能受到影响的人都应有机会在传染病暴发的规划和应对的所有阶段，直接或通过合法代表表达他们的声音。应当设立适宜的交流平台和工具，以促进与卫生当局进行交流。

- 特别脆弱的情况——正如准则 3 中进一步讨论的那样，应当特别注意确保在传染病暴发期间更易受伤害或遭遇不公正待遇的人能够对有关传染病暴发的规划和应对的决策提供建议。公共卫生官员应当认识到这些人可能不信任政府和其他机构，并作出特别努力将他们纳入社区参与计划之中。

- 对不同观点持开放态度——沟通交流的目的应是促进真正的双向对话，而不是仅仅作为一种手段来宣布已经作出的决定。决策者应做好准备，认可和讨论替代方法，并根据他们获得的信息修订其决定。尽早与社区联系，并考虑到所有可能受影响的人的利益，对于建立信任和增强社区参与真正对话的能力方面可发挥重要作用。

- 透明性——透明性的伦理原则要求决策者以语言和文化上适当的言辞公开地解释决策的依据。当必须面对不确定的信息作出决策时，应当明确承认不确定性并将其传达给公众。

- 问责——公众应当知道谁负责制定和实施与疫情暴发应对有关的决策，以及如何能够质疑他们认为不适当的决策。

媒体将在任何传染病暴发的应对中发挥重要作用。因此，重要的是确保媒体能够获得关于该疾病及其管理的准确而及时的信息。政府、非政府组织和学术机构应努力支持媒体在传播风险信息的相关科学概念和技术方面的培训，以免引起不必要的恐慌。对公共卫生部门的员工进行传媒培训也很重要，因为他们可能会与报道公共卫生问题的媒体互动。反过来，媒体有责任提供准确、真实、平衡的报道。这是媒体伦理学的重要组成部分。

3. 特别脆弱的情况

> **要解决的问题：**
> · 在传染病暴发期间，为什么某些个人和群体被认为特别脆弱？
> · 在传染病暴发期间，脆弱性如何影响一个人获得服务的能力？
> · 在传染病暴发期间，脆弱性如何影响一个人分享和接收信息的意愿和能力？
> · 在传染病暴发期间，为什么污名化和歧视特别危险？
> · 在应对传染病的工作中，何种方式可能使脆弱人群承受不成比例的负担，或对资源的需要更大？

在传染病暴发期间，某些个人和群体面临更容易受到伤害或不公正对待。政策制定者和疫情应对人员应制定计划，在疫情暴发前满足这些个人和群体的需要，并在疫情暴发时作出合理努力，确保这些需要得到切实满足。要做到这一点，就需要持续关注社区参与，并在社区代表和政府行动者之间建立活跃的社交网络。

在如何解决个人和群体可能是脆弱的问题时，应当考虑到下列各点：

- 难以获得服务和资源——造成社会脆弱性的许多特征可能使个人难以获得必要的服务。例如，身体残障的人可能有运动障碍，即使短距离出行也很困难或不可能。其他社会脆弱人群可能无法获得安全可靠的交通工具，或负有照料责任使他们难以离开家园。此外，脆弱人群可能无法获得清洁水或蚊帐等必要的资源，以减少蚊媒疾病感染的风险。

- 需要有效的可供选择的沟通策略——某些类型的脆弱性可能会妨碍个人发送或接收信息的能力。沟通障碍可能由多种因素造成，包括但不限于文盲、不熟悉当地或官方语言、视力或听力障碍、社交孤立或缺乏互联网和其他通讯服务。这些障碍使个人难以获得必要的公共卫生信息或充分参加社区的活动。为了克服这些障碍，信息应当以多种形式传递（如广播、短信、广告牌、卡通片），并与主要利益攸关者进行直接的口头交流。卫生行政部门不应假定公众会搜索信息，相反，他们应当主动联系相关人群，无论他们在哪里。

- 污名化和歧视的影响——社会脆弱群体成员经常面临相当大的污名化和歧视，在以恐惧和不信任为特征的突发公共卫生事件中，这种污名化和歧视可能会加剧。负责传染病暴发应对的人员应确保所有个人都得到公平和公正的对待，不论其社会地位或被认为其对社会的"价值"如何。他们还应采取措施防止污名化和社会暴力。

- 疫情暴发应对措施负担不成比例——即使公共卫生措施的设计初衷是最好的，但它们也可能在不经意间给特定人群带来不成比例的负担。例如，要求个人居家隔离检疫可能对那些需要离开家以获得清洁水或食物等基本必需品的人造成灾难性的后果。同样，关闭学校等社会疏散措施可能会给依赖上学获得正常膳食的儿童以及可能没有人照顾儿童的在职父母造成不成比例的负担。

- 对资源的更大需要——对情况特别脆弱的个体，有时需要使用额外的资源来满足其需要。在某些情况下，所需的额外资源相对很小，例如雇用口译员，使得使用少数民族语言的群体成员能够参与社区论坛。在另外一些情况下，可能需要大量的额外资源，例如，移动医疗队集结起来向交通不便的偏远农村地区分发疫苗和开展治疗。在确定是否有必要提供特殊的住宿条件时，考虑费用是正当合理的。实际上，要实现效用最大化的目标，就需要进行这样的评估。然而，尽管保护有限的资源很重要，公平的伦理原则有时可以为向需要更大的人提供更多的资源提供辩护。

- 暴力风险增加——传染病暴发可能加剧社会动荡，增加犯罪，并引发暴力行为，特别是针对少数民族人群或移民等脆弱群体。此外，诸如家庭隔离、检疫隔离或关闭学校和工作设施等公共卫生措施可能引发暴力，特别是针对妇女和儿童的暴力。参与疫情暴发规划和应对行动的官员应做好准备，以应对特定人群会被视为引发传染病暴发或传播的原因而成为攻击目标的可能性；应积极制定策略，以保护这些群体的成员不受暴力风险增加的影响。

4. 稀缺资源的分配

要解决的问题：

· 在传染病暴发期间，需要作出什么类型的资源分配决策？

· 在传染病暴发期间，如何将效用和公平原则应用于分配稀缺资源的决策？

· 在传染病暴发期间，如何将互惠原则应用于分配稀缺资源的决策？

· 在传染病暴发期间，有关资源分配的决策应考虑应用哪些程序？

· 在传染病暴发期间，医疗卫生人员对那些无法获得挽救生命资源的人负有什么义务？

传染病的暴发可能很快使政府和卫生保健系统的能力不堪重负，要求它们对有限资源的分配作出艰难的决定。其中一些决定可能是在分配医疗干预措施的情况下产生的，如医院病床、药物和医疗设备。其他问题可能与应如何利用公共卫生资源的更广泛的问题有关。例如，在监测、健康促进和社区参与等活动之间应当如何分配有限的资源？是否应当将人力资源投入到接触者追踪中，而牺牲对患者的管理？是否应当把有限的资金用于改善水和卫生设施，还是建设检疫隔离设施？

传染病暴发还与其他重要公共卫生问题争夺关注和资源。例如，埃博拉疫情暴发的后果之一是，由于患者人数大量增加以及医疗卫生人员的患病和死亡，一般的医疗卫生服务的可及性下降。结果，在此期间死于结核病、人类免疫缺陷病毒（HIV）和疟疾的人数急剧增加[10]。

各国政府、医疗卫生机构和其他参与应对工作的机构应通过制定在疫情暴发情况下分配稀缺资源的准则，为应对这种情况做好准备。应通过包括广泛利害攸关方参与的、公开而透明的程序来制定这种准则，并应尽可能形成正式书面文件，来确定明确的优先事项和程序。参与制定这些准则的人员应遵循以下考虑：

· 平衡考虑效用和公平——资源分配决策应当以效用和公平的伦理原则为指导。效用原则要求分配资源以实现获益最大化和负担最小化，而公平原则要求注意获益和负担的公平分配。在某些情况下，获益和负担的平等分配可能被认为是公平的，但在另一些情况下，优先分配给境况较差的群体，如穷人、患者或脆弱人群等可能更为公平。完全实现效用和公平并不总是可能的。例如，在大城市设立治疗中心可以提高效用价值，因为它可以用相对较少的资源治疗大量的人。但是，如果这种办法意味着偏远农村地区的孤立社区将获得较少资源时，那么它就可能与公平原则相冲突。解决效用与公平之间的潜在矛盾没有唯一正确的方法；重要的是，决策是基于对当地情况的考虑，其过程是包容和透明的。

- 基于健康相关的考虑来界定效用——为了应用效用的伦理原则，首先必须鉴定将被视为改善福利的结果类型。一般来说，重点应当放在健康相关的受益的分配机制上，无论是根据挽救的生存人总数、挽救的生存年总数，还是根据挽救的质量校正生存年总数来界定。因此，虽然优先考虑疫情暴发至关重要的人员可能是合乎伦理的，但基于与开展社会所需关键服务无关的社会价值考虑，来确定人员优先顺序则是不恰当的。

- 关注脆弱群体的需要——在应用公平的伦理原则时，如准则 3 所述，应特别注意那些最容易受到歧视、污名或孤立的个人和群体。必须特别考虑那些被限制在机构环境中的个人，他们高度依赖他人，可能比生活在社区的人面临更高的感染风险。

- 为在传染病暴发应对中作出贡献的人履行基于互惠的义务——互惠的伦理原则意味着，社会应支持那些为了保护公共利益承担过多负担或风险的人。这一原则使那些冒着自身健康或生命风险而为应对疫情暴发作出贡献的人优先获得稀缺资源。

- 向无法获得挽救生命资源的人提供支持性和姑息性护理——即使不可能向所有能够从中受益的人提供拯救生命的医疗资源，也应努力确保不抛弃任何患者。做到这一点的一种方法是确保有足够的资源用于提供支持性和姑息性护理。

分配原则的应用应考虑到下列因素：

- 一致应用——分配原则应以一致的方式应用于单个机构，以及尽可能一致地应用于各个地区。应制定决策工具，以确保一视同仁，并且确保没有人由于分配计划中未明确识别的社会地位或其他因素而得到更好或更差的对待。在分配方法的选择或应用方面，应当努力避免无意中出现的系统性歧视。

- 解决争端——应当建立机制，解决在分配原则应用方面的分歧。这些机制的设计应当确保任何认为分配原则被不当应用的人有机会参加公正和负责任的审查程序，并有机会发表意见。

- 避免腐败——在传染病暴发期间，如果大量的个人争夺有限的资源，卫生部门的腐败可能会加剧。应当作出努力确保参与实行分配制度的人员不受贿、不行贿、不从事其他腐败活动。

- 责任分离——在可能的范围内，分配原则的解释不应当委托给那些业已存在专业服务关系的临床医生，这些关系造成他们有伦理义务去维护特定患者或群体的利益。相反，应由具有合适资格，并且不存在任何个人或专业服务理由维护一个患者或群体而不是另一个患者或群体的临床医生作出决策。

5. 公共卫生监测

> **要解决的问题：**
>
> · 监测在传染病暴发应对工作中起什么作用？
>
> · 监测活动是否应当接受伦理审查？
>
> · 从事监测活动的实体有哪些义务为所收集的信息保密？
>
> · 在何种情况下，应征求个人同意或给予个人选择不参与监测活动的机会？
>
> · 从事监测活动的人员有何义务向受影响的个人和社区披露他们收集的信息？

　　系统的观察和数据收集是应对措施的基本组成部分，既可以指导对当前疫情暴发的管理，也可以帮助预防和应对未来的疫情暴发。即使这些活动没有被描述为出于监管目的的研究，也应当进行伦理分析，以确保个人信息受到保护，不造成身体、法律、心理和其他的伤害。各国应考虑建立对公共卫生活动进行伦理监督的制度，以符合公共卫生活动的目标、方法、风险和受益，以及这些活动在多大程度上涉及脆弱的个人或群体。无论是否采用这种制度，对公共卫生活动的伦理分析都应符合公认的公共卫生伦理学规范，并由可对其决定负责的个人或实体进行。

　　至少有两个因素使为确保高质量且合乎伦理的监测变得复杂。首先，有关跨管辖区的监测法律可能过于复杂或不一致。其次，监测活动将跨越资源水平不同的管辖区，从而对数据的质量和可靠性造成压力。在传染病暴发期间，这些问题可能会加剧，因此迫切需要仔细规划和开展国际合作。应当解决的具体问题包括以下方面：

· 个人信息的保密——在传染病暴发期间收集的个人信息（包括姓名、地址、诊断、家族史等）未经授权而外泄，会使个人面临重大风险。各国应当确保对这些风险提供充分保护，包括制定法律，以确保对监测活动中所产生的信息保密，并确保严格限制可用于或披露此类信息的目的与最初收集此类信息的目的不同的情况。为研究目的使用和共享非汇总的监测数据必须获得合规设立和经培训的研究伦理委员会的批准。

· 评估普遍参与的重要性——公共卫生监测通常是在强制性的基础上进行的，没有个人拒绝的可能性。如果一个负责任的政府部门认为，为了实现令人信服的公共卫生目的，普遍参与是必要的，那么从公共利益的角度来看，在强制性的基础上收集监测信息在伦理上是恰当的。但是，不应认为监测活动必须始终在强制性的基础上进行。负责设计和批准监测规划的实体应当考虑允许个人选择不参加特定的监测活动的适宜性，并同时考虑所涉及的个人风险的性质和程度，以及允许选择不参加将在多大程度上损害该活动的公共卫生目标。

- 向个人和社区披露信息——无论个人是否被赋予选择不参与监测活动的权利，监测过程都应在透明的基础上进行。至少，个人和社区应当知晓将收集的有关他们的信息的类型，这些信息将用于什么目的，以及收集的信息在什么情况下可能与第三方共享。此外，应可能合理地提供有关监测活动结果的信息。应当认真注意传播这种信息的方式，以使监测对象可能面临的污名化或歧视的风险最小化。

传染病暴发伦理问题管理指南

6. 限制行动自由

要解决的问题：

- 在什么情况下，在传染病暴发期间限制个人行动自由是正当的？
- 对于行动自由受到限制的个人，应保证什么生活条件？
- 对行动自由受到限制的个人还负有什么其他义务？
- 必须建立哪些程序性保护来确保对行动自由的限制得到适当的执行？
- 政策制定者和公共卫生官员有什么义务向公众通报行动自由受到的限制？

对行动自由的限制包括隔离、检疫、旅行劝告或限制，以及以社区为基础的减少人与人之间接触的措施（例如关闭学校或禁止大型聚会）。这些措施通常可以在控制传染病暴发方面发挥重要作用，并且在这种情况下，采取这些措施得到保护社区福利的伦理价值取向的辩护。但是，不应假定这些措施是有效的。事实上，在某些传染病流行的情况下，它们可能对疫情暴发控制作用甚少或毫无作用，甚至可能产生反作用，从而导致对其他控制措施的抵制。此外，所有这些措施都给个人和社区带来重大负担，包括直接限制基本人权，特别是行动自由及和平集会的权利。

鉴于这些考虑，在对下述问题未予以仔细斟酌前，不应对行动自由加以限制：

- 实施限制的正当依据——应根据与国家和国际公共卫生官员磋商后确定的有关疫情暴发的最佳现有证据为依据，作出限制行动自由的决定。除非有合理的依据预期这些限制干预措施将显著减少疾病传播，否则不应实施此类干预措施。应明确说明这些限制措施所依赖的理由，并应根据新出现的有关疫情暴发的科学信息，不断重新评估任何限制措施的适当性。如果施加限制的最初理由不再适用，则应当立即取消限制。

- 限制最少的方式——对行动自由的任何限制应以合理可能的最少限制的方式设计和实施。只有在有充分理由相信较少的限制措施不太可能实现重要的公共卫生目标时，才应实施更严格的限制。例如，自愿合作的要求通常比法律或军事当局执行的公共卫生指令更为可取。同样，在将个人限制在机构内之前，应考虑以家庭为基础的隔离检疫。虽然通常建议对已经出现症状的个人，特别是具有高度传染性的疾病，在设备齐全的医疗机构中隔离，但有时可能适合居家隔离检疫，但条件是：能够组织充分的医疗和后勤支持，家庭护理人员愿意并能够在训练有素的公共卫生人员的监督下采取行动。如果工作量使设施容量不堪重负，则尤应如此。

- 成本——在某些情况下，限制较少的替代方案可能涉及更大的成本。这本身并不能证明采取限制性更大的办法是正当的。但是，可以合理地考虑成本和其他实际制约因素（例如后勤、距离、现有劳动力），以确定在这种情况下，特别是在资源严重紧缺的情况下，一种限制较少的选择是否可行。

- 确保人道条件——对行动自由的任何限制，特别是那些不是自愿的限制，都应得到充分资源的支持，以确保受到限制的人不会承受不当的负担。例如，应确保行动受到限制的个人（无论是限制在家中还是在机构中）能够获得食物、饮用水、卫生设施、住所、衣服和医疗。同样重要的是，要确保个人有足够的物理空间、参与活动的机会以及与亲人和外部世界交流的手段。满足这些需要，对尊重个人尊严和解决个人及其亲人被隔离带来的重大社会心理负担是必不可少的。应建立机制，以最大限度地将暴力（包括性侵犯）和当地疾病传播的风险最小化，特别是当个人被限制在机构环境中或社区受到大规模隔离检疫时。至少，由于接触了与导致疫情相关的病原体而被隔离的人员不应因其受到限制的方式而面临更高的感染风险。（如准则3所述，关于隔离情况和条件的决定应考虑到脆弱群体的需要增加。）

- 解决财务和社会后果——即使是对行动自由的短期限制，也可能对个人、他们的家庭和他们的社区产生重大的甚至可能是毁灭性的财务和社会后果。各国应向因无法经营业务、失业、作物受损，或限制行动自由的其他后果而遭受经济损失的家庭提供援助。在某些情况下，这种支持可能需要在隔离结束后持续一段时间。此外，应当作出努力，支持那些不再需要隔离的个人重新融入社会和职业生活，包括采取措施减少污名化和歧视。

- 正当程序保护——应建立机制，允许自由受到限制的个人对这些限制的适当性、实施方式和实施限制的条件提出质疑。如果在紧急情况下实施这些限制之前无法提供充分的正当程序保护，则应立即提供复审和上诉机制，而不应过度拖延。所有参与限制个人行动自由的决定的人都应对任何滥用权力的行为负责。

- 适用公平——对行动自由的限制应以同样的方式适用于所有对公共卫生构成类似风险的人。因此，不能出于与可能给他人带来风险无关的原因，包括其是否属于任何不受欢迎或受欢迎的社会群体或阶级（例如，由性别、族群或宗教所界定的群体），而使个人受到更多或更少的限制。此外，政策制定者应设法确保限制措施的实施方式不会给社会脆弱群体带来不成比例的负担。

- 沟通和透明性——政策制定者和公共卫生官员应当与社区就任何限制行动自由的问题进行对话，并就如何以负担尽可能少的方式实施限制征求社区成员的意见。他们还应定期向广大公众和那些行动受到限制的人提供关于执行这些措施的最新情况。应当制定沟通策略，以避免对自由受到限制的个人进行污名化，并保护其隐私和机密，特别是在媒体中。

7. 与诊断、治疗和预防传染病的医疗干预有关的义务

要解决的问题：

· 在传染病暴发期间，医疗干预的管理应遵循什么样的质量和安全标准？

· 在传染病暴发期间，患者（或其授权的代理决策者）有哪些权利获得关于医疗干预的风险和受益以及替代方法的信息？

· 在传染病暴发期间，在什么情况下（如果有的话）可以无视个人对诊断、治疗或预防措施的拒绝？

· 在传染病暴发期间，在无视个人拒绝诊断、治疗或预防措施之前，应当提供什么程序性的保障措施？

任何用于诊断、治疗或预防传染病的医疗干预措施都应当符合专业的医学标准，并且达到确保患者安全的可获得的最高水平。各国应当在国际专家的支持下，制定受疫情暴发影响患者的照护和治疗的最低标准。这些标准不仅应当适用于医疗机构，也应当适用于以家庭为基础的照护、社区活动（包括健康教育会议）以及环境净化工作或尸体处理。

在诊断、治疗或预防感染性病原体时，向个人提供医疗干预应当告知其相关的风险、受益和替代方案，正如向其提供其他重要医疗干预时一样。我们的推定是，关于接受何种医疗干预措施（如果有的话）的最终决定权应当属于患者。对于缺乏法律能力为自己作出医疗决策的患者，决策一般应当由合适的授权代理决策者作出，并尽可能获得患者的赞同。

医务人员应当认识到，在某些情况下，拒绝诊断、治疗或预防措施可能从精神上具备决策能力的个人视角看是一种理性的选择。如果患者不愿意接受干预，医生应当与患者进行开放和尊重的对话，仔细关注患者的担忧、感知和情境需要。

在特殊情况下，可能有正当的理由不予理会个人拒绝已被证实是安全和有效的诊断、治疗或预防措施，该措施是公认的医学标准治疗的一部分。决定是否无视患者的拒绝应当基于以下考虑：

· 拟干预措施对公共卫生的必要性——唯有在下列情况下才能无视精神上具备决策能力的个人拒绝诊断、治疗或预防措施：有充分理由相信接受其个人的拒绝将对公众健康构成重大

风险，干预可能会改善这些风险，而且在这种情况下，没有任何其他可行的保护公众健康的措施（包括隔离患者）。

- 拟干预措施存在医疗禁忌——一些可能对人群中多数人构成低风险的干预措施，但会对有特定疾患的个人构成更高的风险。不应当强迫个人接受干预，因为根据他们个人的医疗情况，这些干预会使他们面临重大风险。

- 为不愿接受干预的患者提供干预措施的可行性——在某些情况下，为不愿积极参与干预措施的患者提供干预是不可能的。例如，结核病的标准治疗要求患者定期服药数月，没有患者的合作，期望如此漫长的治疗方案能够顺利完成是不现实的。在这种情况下，保护公共卫生的唯一现实方法也许是隔离患者，直到他或她不再具有传染性，假定以人道的方式这样做是可行的。

- 对社区信任的影响——无视个人对诊断、治疗或预防措施的拒绝，如果导致社区成员对医务人员或公共卫生系统产生不信任，可能会事与愿违。强制实施人们不想要的干预措施的受益应当与危害医疗系统的信任可能造成的伤害相平衡。

在没有给予个人事先通知，且没有给予机会向公正的决策者（例如法院、跨学科审查小组或未参与初始决策的其他实体）提出他或她拒绝的情况下，不得推翻其对诊断、治疗或预防措施的拒绝。干预的提出者有责任证明预期的公共卫生受益可以为推翻个人的选择辩护。解决异议的过程应当符合准则 2 中讨论的原则，以公开、透明的方式进行。

8. 传染病暴发期间的研究

要解决的问题：

- 在传染病暴发期间，研究的适当角色是什么？
- 传染病暴发的情况如何影响研究方案的伦理审查？
- 传染病暴发的情况如何影响研究的知情同意过程？
- 哪些设计方法适合用于传染病暴发期间进行的研究？
- 如何将研究整合入更广泛的疫情暴发应对工作？

在传染病暴发期间，在道德上有义务尽可能多地、尽可能快地了解情况，以便为正在进行的公共卫生应对提供信息，并考虑对正在测试的新干预措施进行适当的科学评价。这种办法也将改进对未来类似疫情暴发的准备工作。履行这一义务要求精心设计和合乎伦理地开展科学研究。除了评价诊断、治疗或预防措施（如疫苗）的临床试验外，其他类型的研究（包括流行病学、社会科学和实施性研究）在降低发病率和死亡率，以及处理暴发所造成的社会和经济后果方面可以发挥关键作用。

在传染病暴发期间进行的研究，其设计和实施应当与其他公共卫生干预措施协同。在任何情况下，研究都不应损害公共卫生对疫情暴发的应对或影响提供适宜的临床医疗服务。所有临床试验必须在合适的临床试验注册中心提前进行注册。

与疫情未暴发时的情况一样，必须确保研究具有科学依据并增加社会价值；风险相对于预期受益是合理的；参与者的选择是公平的，参与是自愿的（在大多数情况下，是遵循明确的知情同意过程的）；参与者的权利和福祉得到充分保护；研究经过充分的独立审查程序。这些国际公认的规范和标准源于有益、尊重人和公正的基本伦理原则。它们适用于涉及人的所有研究领域，无论是生物医学、流行病学、公共卫生或社会科学研究，并在很多国际伦理准则中作了详细解释[11, 12, 13, 14, 15]，所有这些都完全适用于疫情暴发情况。研究中的所有角色，包括研究人员、研究机构、研究伦理委员会、国家监管机构、国际组织和商业赞助商，都有义务确保在疫情暴发情况下遵守这些原则。这样做要求注意以下考量：

- 当地研究机构的作用——当有当地研究人员时，他们应参与疫情暴发有关研究的设计、实施、分析、报告和发表。当地研究人员能够帮助确保研究工作充分响应当地的现实和需要，并确保在不危及紧急应对的情况下有效实施这些研究。让当地研究人员参与国际研究合作也有助于在受影响国家建立长期研究的能力，并促进科学领域中国际公平的价值。

- 解决当地研究伦理审查和科学能力方面的局限性——由于时间限制、缺乏专业知识、资源转用于疫情暴发应对工作或来自公共卫生当局的压力削弱了审查者的独立性，因此在疫情暴发期间，各国参与当地研究伦理审查的能力可能会受到限制。国际组织和非政府组织应当协助当地研究伦理委员会克服这些挑战，例如，通过发起由多个国家的代表参加并由外部专家补充的协作审查。

- 在时效性很强的情况下提供伦理审查——需要立即采取行动以控制传染病的暴发，这可能使我们无法遵守通常的研究伦理审查时间表。国家研究治理体系和国际社会应当预见到这一问题，通过建立机制来确保紧急情况下加快伦理审查，而又不损害伦理审查旨在提供的任何实质性保护。一种选项是授权在疫情暴发条件下对通用的研究方案进行预先审查，然后可以针对特定情境对其进行迅速调整和审查。尽早与当地研究伦理委员会进行讨论和协作有助于确保研究项目是可行的，并有助于当地委员会在疫情实际暴发时有效和高效地审议最终研究方案。

- 将研究整合入更广泛的疫情应对工作之中——国家有关当局和国际组织应当设法协调研究计划，以便确定与更广泛的暴发疫情应对工作相一致的优先事项，并避免不必要的重复研究工作或不同研究中心之间的竞争。如果研究对正在进行的应对工作很重要，研究人员有义务共享所收集的信息作为研究的一部分，例如有关隐匿病例和传播链的信息，或对抗应对措施的信息。共享信息和接收信息的人应当尽可能地保护个人信息的机密性。作为知情同意过程的一部分，研究人员应当告知潜在的参与者在何种情况下他们的个人信息可能与公共卫生当局共享。

- 确保研究不会耗尽与健康相关的重要资源——如果研究会过度占用其他重要的临床和公共卫生的资源，包括人员、设备和医疗设施，则不应进行研究。研究方案应当包括当地能力建设的条款，例如使当地合作者参与进来并对其进行培训，或在可能的情况下留下任何可能有用的工具或资源。

- 面对恐惧和绝望——对传染病暴发典型的恐惧和绝望气氛可能会使伦理委员会或潜在的参与者难以对研究的风险和受益进行客观评估。在一个有大量的人生病和死亡的环境中，任何潜在的干预都可能被认为是比什么都没有好，而不顾实际涉及的风险和潜在的受益如何。负责批准研究方案的人员应当确保，除非有合理的科学依据相信试验性干预可能是安全和有效的，而且风险已经在可能合理的范围内最小化，否则不要启动临床试验。此外，研究者和伦理委员会应认识到，在疫情暴发期间，潜在的参与者可能特别容易产生治疗误解，即错误地认为干预主要是为了直接有利于参与者个人，而不是为将来人们的潜在受益而发展可普遍化的知识。事实上，研究人员自身以及人道主义救援工作者有时可能无法区分从事研究和提供常规临床医疗服务。应当作出努力在可能合理的范围内消除这种治疗误解。尽管作出了这些努力，一些潜在的参与者可能仍然没有充分认识到研究和常规医疗之间的区别，但这本身不应当妨碍他们的参与。

- 应对知情同意的其他障碍——除了恐惧和绝望的影响之外，其他因素也可能会挑战研究人员获取研究知情同意的能力，这些因素包括外国研究人员和当地参与者之间的文化和语言差异，以及被建议隔离或已被隔离的潜在参与者可能与家庭和其他支持系统失去联系，无法拒绝参与研究的邀请。应当尽可能与当地社区协商，制定符合国际研究伦理准则的同意程序，并由当地的招聘人员实施。此外，研究人员应当充分了解当地可获得的医疗、心理和社会支持系统，以便他们能够指导有需要的参与者使用这些服务。在某些情况下，也许有必要建立快速的机制来任命代理决策者，例如在影响认知能力的疾病暴发期间，或当疫情暴发留下成为孤儿的大量儿童时。

- 获得和维持信任——在研究设计和实施过程中，或在披露初步结果时，未能建立和维持社区信任，不仅会阻碍研究的招募和完成，而且还可能妨碍接受任何已被证实有效的干预措施。在研究前、中和后与受影响的社区进行接触，对于建立和维持信任至关重要。在公众对政府的信任很脆弱的环境中，研究人员应当尽可能独立于官方的公共卫生活动。如果政府工作人员自己参与进行研究，他们应当告知参与者这一事实。个人若发现以公共卫生或应急措施的名义进行的不符合伦理的做法，应立即向伦理委员会或其他独立机构报告。

- 选择合适的研究方法——如果研究的设计不能获得有效的结果，那么将研究参与者暴露在风险之下在伦理学上是不可接受的。因此，所有的研究都必须以一种严谨的方法设计和实施。在临床试验中，诸如随机化、安慰剂对照、盲法或设盲等设计要点的适宜性应当根据具体案例加以确定，同时注意数据的科学有效性和参与者所在社区对研究方法的接受程度。在依赖定性方法的研究中，使用诸如焦点小组（该小组的个人保密性无法得到保证）或与受创伤的受害者面谈等方法的潜在受益应与所涉个人的风险和负担相平衡。

- 快速数据共享：正如世界卫生组织先前所认可的，一旦初步结果得到充分的质量控制以供发布，每一位从事与突发公共卫生事件或有可能发展为突发公共卫生事件的紧急事件相关的信息生成工作的研究人员都有基本的道德义务共享初步结果[16]。这些信息应当与公共卫生官员、研究参与者和受影响的人群，以及参与更广泛的国际应对工作的团体共享，不必等待在科学期刊上发表。期刊应促进这一进程，允许研究人员快速传播对公众健康有直接影响的信息，同时不失去随后考虑在期刊上发表的机会。

- 确保研究受益的公平可及——正如现行国际伦理准则所认可的，参与研究的个人和社区应当酌情获得其参与研究所产生的任何受益。研究发起者和东道国应当事先商定各种机制，以确保在研究中发现的任何安全有效的干预措施都将及时提供给当地居民，包括在可行情况下，在监管部门最终批准之前，予以同情使用。

9. 未经证实的干预措施在研究之外的紧急使用

传染病暴发伦理问题管理指南

> **要解决的问题:**
> · 在何种情况下，在传染病暴发期间，在临床试验之外，向患者提供未经证实的干预措施在伦理学上是合适的？
> · 如何确定此类干预措施？
> · 在传染病暴发期间，当在临床试验之外提供未经证实的干预措施时，应当进行何种伦理监督？
> · 如果提供了此类干预措施，应当向个人告知哪些信息？
> · 在临床试验之外实施未经证实的干预措施的人员承担哪些与社区沟通的义务？
> · 在临床试验之外实施未经证实的干预措施的人员承担哪些分享结果的义务？

有许多病原体，对它们没有证实有效的干预措施。对于某些病原体，也许有一些干预措施在实验室和相关动物模型中已显示出具有良好的安全性和有效性，但尚未对人的安全性和有效性进行评价。在正常情况下，这些干预措施经过临床试验的研究，能够产生关于安全性和有效性的可靠证据。然而，在具有高死亡率的疫情暴发背景下，在临床试验之外的紧急情况下为个别患者提供试验性干预措施在伦理上学是合适的，前提是：

1) 没有已证实有效的治疗方法；

2) 不可能立即启动临床研究；

3) 至少可以从实验室或动物研究中获得干预措施的有效性和安全性的初步支持数据，并且在风险－受益分析有利的基础上，具有合适资格的科学咨询委员会已经建议在临床试验之外使用干预措施；

4) 国家相关主管部门和具有合适资格的伦理委员会已批准这种使用；

5) 可获得足够的资源以确保能够使风险最小化；

6) 获得患者的知情同意；以及

7) 对干预措施的紧急使用进行监控，并将结果记录在案，及时与更广泛的医学界和科学界共享。

正如世界卫生组织先前指南中所解释的那样，在这些情况下使用试验性干预措施被称为"监控下紧急使用未注册的试验性干预措施"（monitored emergency use of unregistered and experimental interventions，MEURI）[18]。

MEURI 的伦理基础——MEURI 因尊重患者自主权的伦理原则而得到辩护，即个人有权根据他们个人的价值观、目标和健康状况自行进行风险－受益评估。MEURI 也得到了有益原则的支持——为患者提供可获得的和合理的机会改善他们的病情，包括有理由相信能够减轻极端痛苦和提高生存机会的措施。

MEURI 的科学基础——除非为此目的特别设立的具有合适资格的科学咨询委员会首先建议，否则各国不应当批准 MEURI。该委员会的建议应当建立在对来自实验室、动物和人的干预研究的所有数据进行严格审查的基础之上，以评估在未接受 MEURI 患者所受风险背景下的 MEURI 风险与受益。

MEURI 应遵循与指导临床试验使用未经证实的化合物相同的伦理原则，包括以下内容：

- 伦理监督的重要性——MEURI 是在无法启动临床试验的情况下所采取的例外措施，而不是为了规避对使用未经证实干预措施的伦理监督。因此，应当建立机制来确保 MEURI 接受伦理监督。

- 有效的资源分配——MEURI 不应妨碍或延迟试验产品的临床研究。此外，它不应转移对实施有效的临床医疗和／或公共卫生措施的注意力或资源，这些措施可能对控制疫情暴发至关重要。

- 最小化风险——实施未经证实的干预措施必然涉及风险，其中一些风险在进一步测试之前无法完全理解。然而，任何与干预相关的已知风险都应在可能合理的范围内最小化（例如，在符合卫生的条件下给药；采用与临床试验期间使用的相同安全防范措施，密切监测并可获得紧急药物和设备；以及提供必要的支持性治疗）。唯有根据 GMP（良好的生产规范）生产的试验产品才能用于 MEURI。

- 收集和共享有意义的数据——负责监管 MEURI 的医生与负责监管临床试验的研究人员一样，有同样的道德义务收集所有与干预措施安全性和有效性相关的科学数据。应尽可能汇总所有患者身上通过 MEURI 产生的知识，并与 MEURI 科学咨询委员会、公共卫生当局、该国的医生和研究人员，以及国际医学和科学界进行透明、完整和快速的共享。应当准确地描述信息，不要夸大受益或低估不确定性或风险。

- 知情同意的重要性——应当让获得 MEURI 的个人意识到，干预可能对他们没有受益，甚至可能伤害他们。获取对 MEURI 的知情同意的过程应以文化和语言敏感的方式进行，并强调所告知信息的内容和可理解性，以及患者决定的自愿性。如果患者处于可以作出选择的状态，是否接受未经证实的干预，其最终选择必须取决于患者。如果患者处于无意识状态、认知障碍或病得太重，不能理解信息，则应当从家庭成员或其他授权决策者处获得代理同意。

- 需要社区参与——MEURI 必须对当地的规范和惯例保持敏感。设法确保这种敏感性的一个方法是使用快速的"社区参与团队",以促进对尚未经过临床试验测试的干预措施的潜在受益和风险进行对话。
- 面临资源稀缺时的公平分配——可能无法大量获得符合 MEURI 标准的化合物。在这种情况下,必须就谁接受每次干预作出选择。各国应建立作出这些分配决定的机制,同时考虑到 MEURI 科学咨询委员会的评估和准则 4 中讨论的原则。

10. 快速的数据共享

要解决的问题：

· 为什么在传染病暴发期间快速数据共享至关重要？

· 与快速数据共享相关的关键伦理问题是什么？

数据的收集和共享是日常公共卫生实践的基本组成部分。在传染病暴发期间，由于科学信息的不确定性和不断变化、当地卫生系统应对能力受损，以及跨境合作的作用提升，使得数据共享变得更加紧迫。由于这些理由，"在突发卫生事件中的快速数据共享至关重要"[19]。在伦理学上合适且快速的数据共享能够帮助鉴别病因，预测疾病传播，评价现有和新的治疗方法、对症处理和预防措施，以及指导有限资源的部署。

产生数据的活动包括公共卫生监测、临床研究、个别患者的境遇（包括 MEURI），以及流行病学、定性和环境研究。所有参与这些工作的个人和实体都应当通过及时分享有关的和准确的数据进行合作。如准则 8 所述，应当努力确保快速分享对公共卫生有直接影响的信息而不妨碍该信息随后在科学期刊上发表。

作为正在进行的传染病流行前的准备工作的一部分，各国应审查其有关数据共享的法律、政策和实践，以确保它们能充分保护个人信息的机密性，并能解决其他有关的伦理问题，诸如如何管理偶然的发现，以及处理有关信息所有权或控制权的争端。

11. 传染病暴发期间所收集的生物标本的长期储存

> **要解决的问题：**
>
> · 长期储存传染病暴发期间收集的生物标本有什么受益和风险？
>
> · 参与长期储存传染病暴发期间收集的生物标本的实体，与社区协商有哪些义务？
>
> · 对于长期储存传染病暴发期间收集的生物标本，在什么情况下，应当征得个人同意或给予机会选择不同意？
>
> · 在国内或国际上将生物标本转移到收集机构之外时，应当考虑什么？

传染病暴发期间，在诊断（例如，确定谁感染了或接触了新型病原体）、监测（例如，确定耐药细菌的发病率）或研究（例如，在新的诊断、疫苗或干预措施的临床试验期间）的情境下通常会收集生物样本。这些标本会被送往现场的实验室或国内外的其他实验室进行分析。

在管理传染病暴发期间收集的生物标本为研究人员提供了重要机会，以更好地了解传染病暴发的病原体，并制定诊断、治疗和预防措施，以减轻未来类似疫情暴发的伤害。同时，生物标本的长期储存对个人和社区具有潜在风险。个人面临的风险主要与不想要的个人信息泄露有关。这可以通过保护个人身份的机密性来最小化风险，但是当只有少数人接受检测的情况下，机密性可能很难得到保护。此外，即使个人机密能够得到充分保护，一些个人或社区可能仍然不愿意将其生物标本用于将来的使用，特别是在这种使用不受社区控制的情况下。当标本未经原产国事先的协议同意而转移到国外时，可能会引起特别的关切。解决这些关切需要耗费时间，但很有必要，包括关系建设、咨询和教育，以及建立能够赢得公众信心和信任的政策、措施和制度。

除本指南其他部分讨论的一般原则外，与在传染病暴发期间收集的生物标本的长期储存有关的特殊考虑包括以下几点：

- 提供信息——在请求个人在传染病暴发期间提供生物标本之前，应向他们提供如下信息：有关收集目的，其标本是否会被储存，如果会，他们的标本将来可能会以什么方式被使用。在可行且符合公共卫生目的时，应当征得个人的知情同意，或给予其选择不同意长期储存其标本的机会。如果这些标本有可能以后用于研究目的，征得知情同意尤为重要。

- 社区参与——参与长期储存传染病暴发期间收集的生物标本工作的个人和组织，应当与当地社区的代表就这一过程进行对话。社区代表应当参与制定关于标本未来使用的政策，包括确保公平获得在研究中使用这些标本所产生的任何受益的措施。

- 生物标本的国际共享——有时候有必要在国际上共享生物标本，以进行关键的研究。如果有必要在国际上转移标本，应当建立合适的治理机制和监管制度，以确保标本采集的所在国家的代表参与有关标本使用的决策。国际社会应当努力加强各国在本国境内保存生物标本的能力。

- 材料转移协议——未经正式的材料转移协议，生物标本不应当转移到收集生物标本的国家／地区之外。此类协议应当具体说明转移的目的，证明标本捐赠者的同意是合适的，规定了充分的机密性保护，覆盖标本的物理安全性，要求在未来的研究报告中注明标本原产地，并保证标本的任何后续使用的受益将与提供标本的社区分享。材料转移协议的制定应当包括负责患者医疗和标本采集的人员、受影响社区和患者的代表，以及有关政府官员和伦理委员会。

12. 处理生物学性别和社会性别为基础的差异

> **要解决的问题：**
> · 生物学性别和社会性别如何与传染病暴发有关？
> · 如何将生物学性别和社会性别纳入公共卫生和监测？
> · 与社会性别角色有关的社会和文化习俗如何影响传染病暴发？
> · 在传染病暴发期间应当如何安全地提供合适的生殖卫生保健服务？
> · 在传染病暴发期间，生物学性别和社会性别如何与沟通策略有关？

生物学性别（生物学和生理学特征）和社会性别（社会构建的角色、行为、活动和属性）[20]能够影响传染病暴发的传播、遏制、过程和后果。生物学性别和社会性别差异一直与对感染的易感性、接受的卫生保健水平以及疾病过程和结局相关联[21]。在传染病暴发处理计划和应对工作中处理生物学性别和社会性别的差异要求注意以下几点：

- 将生物学性别和社会性别纳入监测项目——公共卫生监测应当系统地收集关于生物学性别、社会性别和妊娠状况的分类信息，以鉴认不同的风险和传播模式，并监测传染病暴发的任何不同影响，以及用于控制疾病暴发的干预措施。这些信息对孕妇及其后代尤其重要。

- 确保提供高质量的生殖卫生保健服务——不论目前是否怀孕，育龄妇女在传染病暴发期间应享有全面的高质量生殖卫生保健服务。这些服务的组织和提供方式不应当使其使用者被污名化，也不应当使他们面临感染传染病病原体的更大风险。如果有证据表明，某种传染病对孕妇或其胎儿造成特殊风险，则应当将这些风险告知男性和女性，并使其有机会获得安全方法以使风险最小化，同时提供生殖咨询服务。

- 纳入生物学性别和社会性别的研究策略——研究人员应当努力确保研究不会不成比例地偏向特定的性别，并确保怀孕或可能怀孕的妇女不会被不合适地排除在研究参与之外。在疫情暴发期间，对试验性治疗和预防措施的研究应当设法鉴认研究结果中任何与生物学性别和社会性别有关联的差异。

- 注意社会和文化习俗——与社会性别有关的角色和习俗能够影响传染病暴发的所有方面，

包括个人被感染的风险、感染的后果、他们使用卫生服务和其他寻求健康的行为，以及他们易受人际暴力伤害的程度。政策制定者和疫情暴发应对者应当鉴认并应对这些因素，并在可能的情况下利用有关的人类学和社会学研究。

- 对生物学性别和社会性别敏感的沟通策略——负责制定和实施沟通策略的实体应当对个人如何获取和应对与健康相关信息方面存在基于生物学性别和社会性别差异具有敏感性。可能需要使用单独的信息和沟通策略，以便向特定的亚群体（如孕妇或哺乳母亲）提供有关信息。

13. 一线应对工作人员的权利和义务

要解决的问题：

· 在保护参与传染病暴发应对行动的一线工作人员的健康方面有哪些义务？

· 在向参与传染病暴发应对行动的一线工作人员提供物质支持方面有哪些义务？

· 这些义务在多大程度上延伸到工作人员的家庭？

· 在确定个人在传染病暴发期间是否有义务担任一线工作人员时，应当考虑哪些因素？

· 在传染病暴发期间，卫生保健部门的工作人员有哪些特殊义务？

有效的传染病暴发应对措施取决于多种类别的一线工作人员的贡献，其中一些工作人员可能是在志愿的基础上进行工作。这些工作人员经常承担相当大的个人风险来完成他们的工作。在医疗部门内，一线工作人员的范围从直接负责照顾患者的医疗护理专业人员，到传统行医者、救护车司机、实验室工作人员和医院辅助人员。在卫生部门之外，环卫工人、殡葬人员、国内人道主义救援工作者，以及进行接触者追踪的人员也发挥着关键作用。其中一些工作人员可能是社会中最脆弱的成员，他们对自己被要求履行的职责类型几乎没有控制权。在疫情暴发前的规划期间，有必要明确规定一线工作人员的权利和义务，以确保所有行动者都知晓一旦疫情暴发，他们可以合理地预期会发生什么。

具有某些专业资格的工作人员，如医生、护士和葬礼主管人，可能有义务承担一定程度的个人风险，作为其专业或就业承诺的一部分。许多一线工作人员并无此义务，因此他们承担的风险必须被视为超出职责范围（即"超职责"）的。这对于环卫工作人员、殡葬人员和社区卫生工作者来说尤其如此，他们中的许多人可能签订了不稳定的就业合同而没有社会保障，或者在志愿者的基础上工作。

在传染病暴发期间，无论特定个人是否有既存义务承担较高的风险，一旦工作人员承担了这些风险，社会就有互惠的义务提供必要的支持。要履行社会对一线工作人员的互惠义务，至少要求采取以下行动：

• 尽量减少感染的风险——除非向个人提供必要的培训、工具和资源，使风险降到合理可能的程度，否则不应当在传染病暴发期间让他们承担危险的工作任务。这包括关于已知的病原体的性质和感染控制措施的完整和准确的信息，有关当地传染病流行情况的最新信息，以及个人防护装备的提供。应当定期对一线工作人员进行筛查，以尽快发现任何感染情况，以便立即进行医疗处置，并将传染给同事、患者、家人和社区成员的风险降至最低。

- 优先获得医疗保健——应确保生病的一线工作人员、以及通过与工作人员接触而患病的任何直系亲属能够获得合理可得的最高水平的医疗服务。此外，各国应当考虑在疫苗和其他治疗可获得时优先向一线工作人员及其家属提供。

- 合适的薪酬——应当给予一线工作人员公平的工作薪酬。各国政府应当确保及时向公共部门工作人员支付工资，并努力确保私营和非政府部门的行动者向其雇员和承包商履行支付义务。一线工作人员的公平薪酬，包括因在工作中感染而不能履行正常职责期间向其提供的经济支持。

- 支持重新融入社区——一线工作人员可能会遭受污名化和歧视，特别是那些参与不受欢迎措施的人员，例如不按照传统习俗进行的感染控制或埋葬。各国政府应当努力减少受污名化和歧视的风险，并帮助这些工作人员重新融入社区，包括提供就业安排援助和必要时迁移到其他社区。

- 向家庭成员提供援助——应当向需要离开家庭以便履行职责或从疾病中康复的一线工作人员的家庭提供援助。应当向因公殉职的一线工作人员的家属，包括志愿人员或"临时工"，提供死亡津贴。

如上所述，一些工作人员在传染病暴发期间负有职责坚持工作。然而，即使对这些个人来说，承担风险的职责也不是无限的。在确定工作人员承担个人风险的职责范围时，应考虑以下因素：

- 互惠义务——任何以专业或就业为基础的承担个人风险的义务，都取决于社会履行它前面所述的对工作人员的互惠义务。如果不履行互惠义务，就不能正当地要求一线工作人员承担对自己和家人造成重大伤害的风险。

- 风险和受益——不应当要求一线工作人员将自己暴露于与其努力可能实现的公共卫生受益不成比例的风险之中。

- 公平和透明性——负责为一线工作人员分配具体任务的实体应当确保以公平的方式在个人和职业类别之间分配风险，并确保分配工作人员的程序尽可能透明。

- 不参与的后果——应当告知一线工作人员他们被要求承担的风险。在可能的情况下，应在书面就业协议中阐明对他们的期望。不愿意接受合理风险和工作分配的工作人员可能会受到职业影响（例如，失去工作），但额外的处罚（如罚款或监禁）通常是没有依据的。负责评估不参与后果的人应当认识到，工作人员有时可能需要在其他义务（如对家庭的责任）和与工作有关的责任之间取得平衡。

卫生保健部门工作人员的其他义务：

除上述问题外，卫生保健部门的工作人员在传染病暴发期间对社区负有义务，包括以下内容：

- 参与公共卫生监测和报告工作——在卫生部门工作的人员有义务参与有组织的措施，以应对传染病暴发，包括公共卫生监测和报告。卫生保健工作人员应当以与正当的公共卫生利益相容的方式，最大程度地保护患者信息的机密性。

- 向公众提供准确的信息——在传染病暴发期间，公共卫生官员负有的主要责任是传达有关疫情暴发病原体的信息，包括病原体如何传播，如何预防感染，以及哪些治疗或预防措施可能有效。负责设计沟通策略的人应当预见并应对误报、夸大和不信任，并应当在不隐瞒关键信息的前提下，对导致污名化和歧视相关风险因素的信息，设法使其风险最小化。如果患者或普通民众向卫生部门的工作人员询问有关疫情暴发的医疗问题，他们不应当散布未经证实的谣言或怀疑，并确保他们提供的信息来源可靠。

- 避免剥削——一种威胁生命的疾病迅速蔓延，在没有已证实的有效治疗的情况下，绝望的个人可能愿意尝试提供的任何干预措施，而不顾其预期的风险或受益如何。医务人员有义务不去利用个人的脆弱性，提供没有合理的根据让人相信潜在受益大于不确定性和风险的治疗或预防措施。这一义务并不排除合理使用未经证实的试验性干预措施，这与准则 9 中阐述的准则相一致。

14. 派遣外国人道主义救援人员时的伦理问题

> **要解决的问题：**
> · 当传染病暴发时，派遣外国救援工作人员执行任务会出现什么伦理问题？
> · 发起组织在使外国救援人员为其任务做好充分准备方面负有哪些义务？
> · 发起组织在派遣条件方面有哪些义务？
> · 发起组织与当地官员协调方面有哪些义务？
> · 外国救援人员在派遣前、中、后有什么义务？

在传染病暴发时派遣工作人员的外国政府和人道主义救援组织对工作人员本人和受影响的社区都负有伦理义务。这些义务包括以下方面：

- 与当地官员协调——外国政府和外部人道主义救援组织应当在就救援人员的角色和责任与当地官员讨论并达成协议后派遣工作人员，如果无法做到这一点，则应当与类似世界卫生组织的国际组织讨论并达成协议。在特定区域工作的人员应向当地政府登记为外国紧急医疗队（Emergency Medical Team，EMT），并与他们及当地政府进行持续讨论，以澄清和协调他们的角色和责任，并解决实践标准中的任何差异问题。应当努力与地方当局和医务人员进行协调，以确保外国机构不会从其他基本服务中过度占用资源。

- 派遣外国救援工作人员执行任务的公平性——只有在能够提供当地无法充分获得的必要服务的情况下才应当派遣外国救援工作人员。派遣外国卫生工作人员时，应考虑到他们的相关技能和知识，以及他们的语言和文化能力，以实现任务目标，理解受影响的社区并与之进行交流。仅仅为了满足他们个人或专业的助人愿望而派遣不合格或不必要的工作人员是不合适的（所谓的"灾难旅游"）。

- 明确派遣条件——应当向外国救援工作人员提供关于派遣计划的期望和风险的全面信息，以便他们能够就是否有能力作出适当贡献作出知情的决定。此外，应当清楚地告知外国救援工作人员他们的派遣条件，包括他们生病时可期望的医疗水平、在何种情况下将被遣返、可得的保险，以及如果生病或死亡是否将给予其家属救济金。

- 提供必要的培训和资源——必须为救援人员提供合适的培训、准备和装备，以确保他们能够以切实可行的最低风险有效地执行其任务。培训应包括社会心理和沟通技能的准备，以及了解和尊重当地文化和传统。在当地活动期间和完成任务后，管理者和发起组织有义务向工作人员提供充分的支持和指导。这应当包括应对具有挑战性的伦理问题（如资源分配决策，分级诊疗和不平等）的培训和资源。

- 确保救援人员的安全——派遣外国救援工作人员的组织有义务采取一切必要措施确保这些工作人员的安全，特别是在危机情况下；这项义务包括采取措施，以减少暴露于传染性病原体、污染和暴力的风险。必须建立清晰的权力链以提供监督和持续的建议。个人对所分派的职责有异议，应有机会根据其工作所在组织的规范提出复议和上诉。

救援工作人员对患者、受影响的社区、他们的发起组织和他们自己也有伦理义务。除了本指南其他部分所述的义务外，外国救援工作人员的义务还包括以下方面：

- 充分的准备——救援工作者应当参加所提供的任何培训。如果他们认为他们已经接受的培训不充分，则应当将他们的关切提请他们的组织管理人员注意。在危机期间和资源匮乏的地区部署的外国救援工作人员，应当仔细考虑他们是否准备好应对可能导致道德和心理困扰的伦理问题。

- 遵守分派的角色和责任——救援工作者应当了解他们被要求承担的角色和责任，除非在最极端的情况下，否则不应当从事他们未经授权执行的任务。此外，他们应向其发起组织和当地官员提供清晰和及时的信息，并应当了解如果他们超越了已授权执行的任务，他们不仅将在自己的组织内承担责任，而且将根据适用的当地标准和法律承担责任。

- 注意合适的感染控制措施——救援工作者应保持警惕，遵守感染控制措施，以保护自己和防止疾病的进一步传播。救援工作者应当在服务前、服务期间和服务之后，遵循建议的规程监测症状并报告其健康状况（包括可能的怀孕）。

参考文献

1. Resolution WHA58.3. Revision of the International Health Regulations. In: Fifty-eighth World Health Assembly, Geneva, 16–25 May 2005. Resolutions and decisions, annex. Geneva: World Health Organization; 2005 (WHA58/2005/REC/1; http://apps.who.int/gb/ ebwha/pdf_files/WHA58-REC1/english/A58_2005_REC1-en.pdf, accessed 23 July 2016).

2. Addressing ethical issues in pandemic influenza planning: Discussion papers. Geneva: World Health Organization; 2008 (WHO/HSE/EPR/GIP/2008.2, WHO/IER/ETH/2008.1; http://apps.who.int/iris/ bitstream/10665/69902/1/WHO_IER_ETH_2008.1_eng.pdf?ua=1, accessed 23 July 2016).

3. Guidance on ethics of tuberculosis prevention, care and control. Geneva: World Health Organization; 2010 (WHO/HTM/TB/2010.16, http://apps.who.int/iris/ bitstream/10665/44452/1/9789241500531_ eng.pdf?ua=1, accessed 23 July 2016).

4. Ethics of using convalescent whole blood and convalescent plasma during the Ebola epidemic. Geneva: World Health Organization; 2015 (WHO/HIS/KER/GHE/15.1; http://apps.who.int/iris/bitstream/10665/161912/1/WHO_HIS_KER_GHE_15.1_eng. pdf?ua=1&ua=1, accessed 23 July 2016).

5. Ethical considerations for use of unregistered interventions for Ebola viral disease. Geneva: World Health Organization; 2014 (WHO/HIS/KER/GHE/14.1, http://apps.who. int/iris/bitstream/10665/130997/1/WHO_HIS_KER_GHE_14.1_eng.pdf?ua=1, accessed 23 July 2016).

6. Becker L. Reciprocity, justice, and disability. Ethics. 2005;116(1):9–39.

7. Dawson A, Jennings B. The place of solidarity in public health ethics. Public Health Reviews. 2012;34(1):65–79.

8. Siracusa Principles on the Limitation and Derogation Provision in the International Covenant on Civil and Political Rights. Geneva: American Association for the International Commission of Jurists; 1985 (http://icj.wpengine.netdna-cdn.com/wp-content/uploads/1984/07/Siracusaprinciples-ICCPR-legal-submission-1985-eng.pdf, accessed 23 July 2016).

9. United Nations Economic and Social Council. General Comment No. 14: The right to Highest Attainable Standard of Health (Art. 12 of the International Covenant on Economic, Social and Cultur-

al Rights). New York: United Nations Committee on Economic, Social and Cultural Rights (E/C. 12/2000/4 – 2000; www1.umn.edu/ humanrts/gencomm/escgencom14.htm, accessed 23 July 2016).

10. Parpia AS, Ndeffo-Mbah ML, Wenzel NS, Galvani AP. Effects of response to the 2014–2015 Ebola outbreak on deaths from malaria, HIV/AIDS, and tuberculosis, West Africa. Emerg Infect Dis. 2016;22(3) (http://dx.doi.org/10.3201/eid2203.150977, accessed 23 July 2016).

11. Declaration of Helsinki – Ethical principles for medical research involving human subjects, revised October 2013 Ferney-Voltaire: World Medical Association; 2013 (www.wma.net/ en/30publications/10policies/b3/index.html, accessed 23 July 2016).

12. International ethical guidelines for biomedical research involving human subjects. Geneva: Council for International Organizations of Medical Sciences; 2002 (www.cioms. ch/publications/guidelines/ guidelines_nov_2002_blurb.htm, accessed 23 July 2016).

13. Standards and operational guidance for ethics review of health-related research with human participants. Geneva: World Health Organization; 2011 (www.who.int/ethics/ publications/9789241502948/ en/, accessed 23 July 2016).

14. Ethics in epidemics, emergencies and disasters: Research, surveillance and patient care. Geneva: World Health Organization; 2015 (who.int/ethics/publications/epidemicsemergencies-research/en/, accessed 23 July 2016).

15. Research ethics in international epidemic response. Geneva: World Health Organization; 2009 (WHO/ HSE/GIP/ITP/10.1; www.who.int/ethics/gip_research_ethics_.pdf, accessed 23 July 2016).

16. Developing global norms for sharing data and results during public health emergencies. Geneva: World Health Organization; 2015 (www.who.int/medicines/ebola-treatment/ blueprint_phe_data-share-results/en/, accessed 23 July 2016).

17. Overlapping publications. International Committee of Medical Journal Editors (www. icmje.org/recommendations/browse/publishing-and-editorial-issues/overlappingpublications.html, accessed 23 July 2016).

18. Ethical issues related to study design for trials on therapeutics for Ebola Virus Disease. 2014. Report of the WHO Ethics Working Group meeting, 20–21 October 2014. Geneva: World Health Organization; 2014 (WHO/HIS/KER/GHE/14.2; http://apps.who.int/iris/ bitstream/10665/137509/1/WHO_HIS_KER_GHE_14.2_eng.pdf, accessed 23 July 2016).

19. Dye C, Bartolomeos K, Moorthy V, Kieny MP. Data sharing in public health emergencies: a call to researchers. Bull World Health Organ. 2016;1:94(3):158. doi: 10.2471/ BLT.16.170860 (www.who.int/ bulletin/volumes/94/3/16-170860.pdf?ua=1).

20. Gender, women and health. In: WHO [website]. Geneva: World Health Organization (http://apps.who. int/gender/whatisgender/en/, accessed 23 July 2016).

21. Addressing sex and gender in epidemic-prone infectious diseases. Geneva: World Health Organization; 2007 (www.who.int/csr/resources/publications/SexGenderInfectDis.pdf)

传染病暴发伦理问题管理指南

附件1：制定《传染病暴发伦理问题管理指南》参照的伦理指南文件

世界卫生组织指导文件

Addressing ethical issues in pandemic influenza planning: Discussion papers. Geneva: World Health Organization; 2008 (WHO/HSE/EPR/GIP/2008.2, WHO/IER/ETH/2008.1; http://apps. who.int/iris/bitstream/10665/69902/1/WHO_IER_ETH_2008.1_eng.pdf?ua=1).

Ethical considerations for use of unregistered interventions for Ebola viral disease. Report of an advisory panel to WHO. Geneva: World Health Organization; 2014 (WHO/HIS/KER/ GHE/14.1; http://apps.who.int/iris/bitstream/10665/130997/1/WHO_HIS_KER_GHE_14.1_ eng.pdf?ua=1).

Ethical considerations in developing a public health response to pandemic influenza. Geneva: World Health Organization; 2007 (WHO/CDS/EPR/GIP/2007.2; http://www.who.int/ csr/resources/publications/WHO_CDS_EPR_GIP_2007_2c.pdf?ua=1).

Ethical issues related to study design for trials on therapeutics for Ebola virus disease. WHO Ethics Working Group Meeting, 20–21 October 2014. Geneva: World Health Organization; 2014 (WHO/HIS/KER/GHE/14.2; http://apps.who.int/iris/bitstream/10665/137509/1/WHO_ HIS_KER_GHE_14.2_eng.pdf?ua=1).

Ethics of using convalescent whole blood and convalescent plasma during the Ebola epidemic: Interim guidance for ethics review committees, researchers, national health authorities and blood transfusion services. Geneva: World Health Organization; 2015 (http://apps.who.int/iris/bitstream/10665/161912/1/WHO_HIS_KER_GHE_15.1_eng. pdf?ua=1&ua=1).

Ethics in epidemics, emergencies and disasters: Research, surveillance and patient care: Training manual. Geneva: World Health Organization; 2015 (http://apps.who.int/iris/ bitstre am/10665/196326/1/9789241549349_eng.pdf?ua=1).

Guidance on ethics of tuberculosis prevention, care and control. Geneva: World Health Organization;

2010 (http://apps.who.int/iris/bitstream/10665/44452/1/9789241500531_ eng.pdf?ua=1).

Research ethics in international epidemic response: WHO Technical Consultation. Geneva: World Health Organization; 2009 (www.who.int/ethics/gip_research_ethics_.pdf).

Standards and operational guidance for ethics review of health-related research with human participants. Geneva: World Health Organization; 2011 (http://apps.who.int/iris/ bitstre am/10665/44783/1/9789241502948_eng.pdf?ua=1&ua=1).

国家指导 / 意见文件

Allocation of ventilators in an influenza pandemic: Planning document. New York State Task Force on Life and the Law; 2007 (www.cidrap.umn.edu/sites/default/files/public/ php/196/196_guidance.pdf).

Altevogt BM, Stroud C, Hanson S, Hanfling D, Gostin LO, editors. Guidance for establishing crisis standards of care for use in disaster situations: A letter report. Washington: National Academies Press; 2009 (www.nap.edu/read/12749/chapter/1).

Ethical issues raised by a possible influenza pandemic. Opinion No. 106. Paris: National Consultative Ethics Committee for Health and Life Sciences; 2009 (www.ccne-ethique.fr/ sites/default/ files/publications/avis_106_anglais.pdf).

Ethics and Ebola: Public health planning and response. Washington DC: Presidential Commission for the Study of Bioethical Issues.; 2015 (http://bioethics.gov/sites/default/files/ Ethics-and-Ebola_ PCSBI_508.pdf).

Ethical guidelines in Pandemic Influenza - Recommendations of the Ethics Subcommittee of the Advisory Committee to the Director, United States Centers for Disease Control and Prevention. Ethical guidelines in pandemic influenza. Atlanta: Centers for Disease Control and Prevention; 2007 (www.cdc. gov/od/science/integrity/phethics/docs/panflu_ethic_ guidelines.pdf).

Ethics Subcommittee of the Advisory Committee to the Director, United States Centers for Disease Control and Prevention. Ethical guidance for public health emergency preparedness and response: Highlighting ethics and values in vital public health service. Atlanta: Centers for Disease Control and Prevention; 2008 (www.cdc.gov/od/science/integrity/phethics/docs/ white_paper_final_for_ website_2012_4_6_12_final_for_web_508_compliant.pdf).

Ethics Subcommittee of the Advisory Committee to the Director, United States Centers for Disease Control and Prevention. Ethical considerations for decision making regarding allocation of mechanical ventilators during a severe influenza pandemic or other public health emergency. Atlanta: Centers for Disease Control and Prevention; 2011 (www.cdc. gov/about/pdf/advisory/ventdocument_release.pdf).

Integrated national avian and pandemic influenza response plan, 2007–2009. In: Avian Influenza and the Pandemic Threats: Nigeria. Geneva: United Nations System Influenza Coordination Office (http://un-influenza.org/?q=content/Nigeria).

National Advisory Board on Health Care Ethics. Ethical considerations related to preparedness for a pandemic. Helsinki: Ministry of Social Affairs and Health; 2005 (http:// etene.fi/documents/1429646/ 1561478/2005+Statement+on+ethical+considerations+relate d+to+preparedness+for+a+pandemic.pdf/ fc3f2412-acfc-4685-b427-ca710a43c103).

National Ethics Advisory Committee. Getting through together: Ethical values for a pandemic. Wellington: Ministry of Health; 2007 (https://neac.health.govt.nz/system/files/ documents/publications/ getting-through-together-jul07.pdf).

Notes on the interim US guidance for monitoring and movement of persons with potential Ebola virus exposure. Atlanta GA: Centers for Disease Control and Prevention; 2016 (www. cdc.gov/vhf/ebola/ exposure/monitoring-and-movement-of-persons-with-exposure.html).

Pandemic Influenza Ethics Initiative Workgroup. Meeting the challenge of pandemic influenza: Ethical guidance for leaders and health care professionals in the veterans health administration. Washington DC: National Center for Ethics in Health Care, Veterans Health Administration; 2010 (www.ethics.va.gov/docs/pandemicflu/Meeting_the_Challenge_of_ Pan_Flu-Ethical_Guidance_ VHA_20100701.pdf).

Responding to pandemic influenza: The ethical framework for policy and planning. London: Department of Health; 2007 (www.gov.scot/Resource/Doc/924/0054555.pdf).

Stand on guard for thee: Ethical considerations in preparedness planning for pandemic influenza. Toronto: University of Toronto Joint Centre for Bioethics; 2005 (www.jcb. utoronto.ca/people/documents/ upshur_stand_guard.pdf).

Swiss Federal Office of Public Health. Swiss Influenza Pandemic Plan. Bern; 2013 (www.bag. admin.ch/influenza/01120/01132/10097/10104/index.html?lang=en&download= NHzLpZeg7t,lnp6I0NT U042l2Z6ln1ad1IZn4Z2qZpnO2Yuq2Z6gpJCGenx6gWym162epYb g2c_JjKbNoKSn6A--).

Venkat A, Wolf L, Geiderman JM, Asher SL, Marco CA, McGreevy J et al. Ethical issues in the response to Ebola virus disease in US emergency departments: a position paper of the American College of Emergency Physicians, the Emergency Nurses Association and the Society for Academic Emergency Medicine. J Emerg Nurs. 2015; Mar;41(2):e5-e16. doi: 10.1016/j.jen.2015.01.012 (www.ncbi.nlm.nih. gov/pubmed/25770003).

附件 2： 参加制定《传染病暴发伦理问题管理指南》会议的人员

小组讨论：使用未经注册的干预措施治疗埃博拉病毒病的伦理考量，世界卫生组织，日内瓦，2014 年 8 月 11 日

顾问

Dr Juan Pablo Beca, Professor, Bioethics Center, Universidad del Desarrollo, Chile

Dr Helen Byomire Ndagije, Head, Drug Information Department, Ugandan National Drug Authority, Uganda

Dr Philippe Calain (Chair), Senior Researcher, Unit of Research on Humanitarian Stakes and Practices, Médecins Sans Frontières, Switzerland

Dr Marion Danis, Head, Ethics and Health Policy and Chief, Bioethics Consultation Service, National Institutes of Health, United States of America

Professor Jeremy Farrar, Director, Wellcome Trust, United Kingdom

Professor Ryuichi Ida, Chair, National Bioethics Advisory Committee, Japan

Professor Tariq Madani, infectious diseases physician and clinical academic researcher, Saudi Arabia

Professor Michael Selgelid, Director, Centre for Human Bioethics, Monash University, Australia

Professor Peter Smith, Professor of Tropical Epidemiology, London School of Tropical Medicine and Hygiene, United Kingdom

Ms Jeanine Thomas, Patient Safety Champion, United States of America

Professor Aisssatou Touré, Head, Immunology Department, Institut Pasteurde Dakar,Senegal

Professor Ross Upshur, Chair in Primary Care Research; Professor, Department of Family and Community Medicine and Dalla Lana School of Public Health, University of Toronto; Canada

资源提供者

Dr Daniel Bausch, Head, Virology and Emerging Infections Department, US Naval Medical Research Unit No. 6, Peru

Professor Luciana Borio, Assistant Commissioner for Counterterrorism Policy; Director, Office of Counterterrorism and Emerging Threats, Food and Drug Administration, United States of America

Dr Frederick Hayden, Professor of Clinical Virology and Professor of Medicine, University of Virginia School of Medicine, United States of America

Dr Stephan Monroe, Deputy Director, National Centre for Emerging and Zoonotic Infectious Diseases, Centers for Disease Control and Prevention, United States of America

世界卫生组织秘书处

世界卫生组织总部，瑞士日内瓦

Dr Margaret Chan, Director-General

Dr Marie-Paule Kieny, Assistant Director-General, Health Systems and Innovation

Dr Marie-Charlotte Bouesseau, Ethics Advisor, Service Delivery and Safety

Dr Pierre Formenty, Scientist, Control of Epidemic Diseases, Department of Pandemic and Epidemic Diseases

Dr Margaret Harris, Communication Officer, Department of Pandemic and Epidemic Diseases

Mr Gregory Hartl, Coordinator, Department of Communications

Dr Rüdiger Krech, Director, Health Systems and Innovation

Dr Andreas Reis, Technical Officer, Global Health Ethics, Department of Knowledge, Ethics and Research

Dr Cathy Roth, Adviser, Office of the Assistant Director-General, Health Systems and Innovation

Dr Vasee Sathyamoorthy, Technical Officer, Initiative for Vaccine Research, Department of Immunization, Vaccines and Biologicals

Dr Abha Saxena, Coordinator, Global Health Ethics, Department of Knowledge, Ethics and Research

Dr David Wood, Coordinator, Technologies Standards and Norms, Department of Essential Medicines and Health Products

世界卫生组织区域办事处

Dr Marion Motari, Partnership and Resource Mobilization, Regional Office for Africa, Brazzaville, Congo

Dr Martin Ota, Medical Officer, Health Information and Knowledge Management, Regional Office for Africa, Brazzaville, Congo

Dr Carla Saenz, Bioethics Advisor, Regional Office for the Americas, Washington DC, United States of America

关于潜在埃博拉疗法和疫苗的磋商：世界卫生组织伦理工作组会议，日内瓦，2014 年 9 月 3 日

参加者

Professor Clement Adebamowo, Chair, National Research Ethics Committee, Nigeria Dr Philippe Calain, Senior Researcher, Unit of Research on Humanitarian Stakes and Practices, Médecins Sans Frontières, Switzerland

Dr Marion Danis, Head, Ethics and Health Policy and Chief, Bioethics Consultation Service, National Institutes of Health, United States of America

Professor Jeremy Farrar, Director, Wellcome Trust, United Kingdom

Professor Jennifer Gibson, Sun Life Financial Chair in Bioethics; Director, Joint Centre for Bioethics; and Associate Professor, Institute of Health Policy, Management and Evaluation, University of Toronto, Canada

Ms Robinah Kaitiritimba, Patient Representative (community representative, Makerere University Institutional Review Boards; Uganda National Health Consumers' Organisation), Uganda

Dr Bocar Kouyate, Special Advisor to the Minister of Health (former Chair of National Ethics Committee), Burkina Faso Professor Cheikh Niang, Université Cheikh Anta Diop, Senegal

Professor Michael Selgelid,Director, Centre for Human Bioethics, Monash University, Australia

Professor Oyewale Tomori (Chair), President, Nigeria National Academy of Sciences, Nigeria

Dr Aissatou Touré (Co-Chair), Head, Immunology Department, Institut Pasteur de Dakar and Member, National Ethics Committee, Senegal

世界卫生组织秘书处

世界卫生组织总部，瑞士日内瓦

Dr Andreas Reis, Technical Officer, Global Health Ethics, Department of Knowledge, Ethics and Research

Dr Abha Saxena, Coordinator, Global Health Ethics, Department of Knowledge, Ethics and Research

世界卫生组织区域办事处

Dr Carla Saenz, Bioethics Advisor, Regional Office for the Americas, Washington DC, United States of America

与试验治疗研究设计相关的伦理问题，世界卫生组织，日内瓦，2014 年 10 月 20 日至 21 日

伦理工作组

Professor Arthur Caplan, Drs William F and Virginia Connolly Mitty; Director, Division of Medical

Ethics, New York University Langone Medical Center's Department of Population Health, United States of America

Dr Clare Chandler, Senior Lecturer, Medical Anthropology, Department of Global Health and Development, London School of Hygiene and Tropical Medicine, United Kingdom

Dr Alpha Ahmadou Diallo, Administrator, National Ethics Committee, Ministry of Health and Public Hygiene, Guinea

Dr Amar Jesani, Independent Researcher and Teacher, Bioethics and Public Health; Editor, Indian Journal of Medical Ethics; Visiting Professor, Centre for Ethics, Yenepoya University, India

Dr Dan O'Connor, Head, Medical Humanities, Wellcome Trust, United Kingdom

Dr Lisa Schwartz, Arnold L. Johnson Chair in Health Care Ethics, McMaster Ethics in Healthcare, McMaster University, Canada

Professor Michael Selgelid, Director, Centre for Human Bioethics, Monash University, Australia

Dr Paulina Tindana, Ethicist and Senior Researcher, Navrongo Health Research Centre, Ghana

Professor Ross Upshur, Chair in Primary Care Research; Professor, Department of Family and Community Medicine and Dalla Lana School of Public Health, University of Toronto, Canada

邀请参加者

Dr Enrica Alteri, Head, Human Medicines Evaluation Division, European Medicines Agency, United Kingdom

Dr Nicholas Andrews, Statistics Modelling and Economics Department, Centre for Infectious Disease Surveillance and Control, Public Health England, United Kingdom

Professor Oumou Younoussa Bah-Sow, Head of Pneumophtisiology, Ignace Deen National Hospital, Guinea

Dr Luciana Borio, Assistant Commissioner for Counterterrorism Policy; Director, Office of Counterterrorism and Emerging Threats, Food and Drug Administration, United States of Ameria

Dr Jacob Thorup Cohn; Vice President, Governmental Affairs, Bavarian Nordic, Denmark

Dr Edward Cox, Director, Office of Antimicrobial Products, Office of New Drugs Center for Drug Evaluation and Research, Food and Drug Administration, Silver Spring MD, United States of America

Dr Nicolas Day, Director, Thailand/Laos Wellcome Trust Major Overseas Programme Mahidol-Oxford Tropical Medicine Research Unit, Thailand

Dr Matthias Egger, Professor, Clinical Epidemiology, Department of Social Medicine, University of Bristol, United Kingdom; Epidemiology and Public Health, Institute for Social and Preventive Medicine, University of Bern, Switzerland

Dr Elizabeth Higgs, Global Health Science Advisor, Office of the Director, Division of Clinical Research, National Institute of Allergy and Infectious Diseases, National Institutes of Health, United

States of America

Dr Nadia Khelef, Senior Advisor, Global Affairs, Institut Pasteur, France

Professor Trudie Lang, Lead Professor, Global Health Network, Nuffield Department of Medicine, University of Oxford, United Kingdom

Dr Matthew Lim, Senior Advisor, Global Health Security, Department of Health and Human Services, United States of America

Professor Ira Longini, Professor of Biostatistics, Department of Biostatistics, College of Public Health and College of Medicine, University of Florida, United States of America

Colonel Scott Miller, Director, Infectious Disease Clinical Research Program, Department of Preventive Medicine, Uniformed Services University, United States of America

Ms Adeline Osakwe, Head, National Pharmacovigilance Centre, National Agency for Food and Drug Administration and Control, Nigeria

Ms Virginie Pirard, Member, Belgian Advisory Committee on Bioethics; Ethics Advisor, Institut Pasteur, France

Dr Micaela Serafini, Medical Director, Médecins Sans Frontières, Switzerland

Mr Jemee Tegli, Institutional Review Board Administrator, University of Liberia–Pacific Institute for Research and Evaluation Institutional Review Board, Liberia

Dr Gervais Tougas, Representative, International Federation of Pharmaceutical Manufacturers & Associations, Chief Medical Officer, Novartis, Switzerland

Dr Johan van Griensven, Department of Clinical Sciences, Institute of Tropical Medicine, Belgium

Professor John Whitehead, Emeritus Professor, Department of Mathematics and Statistics, Fylde College, Lancaster University, United Kingdom

世界卫生组织秘书处

Dr Marie-Paule Kieny, Assistant Director-General, Health Systems and Innovation

Dr Marie-Charlotte Bouesseau, Advisor, Department of Service Delivery and Safety

Dr Vânia de la Fuente-Núñez,Technical Officer, Global Health Ethics, Department of Knowledge, Ethics and Research

Dr Martin Friede, Scientist, Public Health, Innovation and Intellectual Property, Department of Essential Medicines and Health Products

Ms Marisol Guraiib, Technical Officer, Global Health Ethics, Department of Knowledge, Ethics and Research

Ms Corinna Klingler, Intern, Global Health Ethics, Department of Knowledge, Ethics and Research

Dr Selena Knight, Intern, Global Health Ethics, Department of Knowledge, Ethics and Research

Dr Nicola Magrini, Scientist, Policy, Access and Use, Department of Essential Medicines and Health

Products

Dr Cathy Roth, Adviser, Office of the Assistant Director-General, Health Systems and Innovation

Dr Vasee Sathiyamoorthy, Technical Officer, Initiative for Vaccine Research, Department of Immunization, Vaccines and Biologicals

Dr Abha Saxena, Coordinator, Global Health Ethics, Department of Knowledge, Ethics and Research

Dr David Wood, Coordinator, Technologies, Standards and Norms, Department of Essential Medicines and Health Products

为流行病期间的公共卫生应对措施（包括进行相关研究）制定伦理准则，爱尔兰都柏林，2015 年 5 月 25 日至 26 日

参加者

Dr Annick Antierens, Manager, Investigational Platform for Experimental Ebola Products, Médecins Sans Frontières, Switzerland

Dr Philippe Calain, Senior Researcher, Unit of Research on Humanitarian Stakes and Practices, Médecins Sans Frontières, Switzerland

Dr Edward Cox, Director, Office of Antimicrobial Products, Food and Drug Administration, United States of America

Professor Heather Draper, Professor of Biomedical Ethics, University of Birmingham, United Kingdom

Dr Sarah Edwards, Senior Lecturer in Research Ethics and Governance, University College London, United Kingdom

Professor Jónína Einarsdóttir, Medical Anthropology, School of Social Sciences, University of Iceland, Iceland

Professor Jeremy Farrar, Director, Wellcome Trust, United Kingdom

Dr Margaret Fitzgerald, Public Health Specialist, Irish Health Service Executive, Ireland

Dr Gabriel Fitzpatrick, Médecins Sans Frontières, Ireland

Ms Lorraine Gallagher, Development Specialist, Irish Aid, Department of Foreign Affairs, Ireland

, Sun Life Financial Chair in Bioethics; Director, Joint Centre for Bioethics; Associate Professor, Institute of Health Policy, Management and Evaluation, University of Toronto, Canada

Professor Frederick G Hayden, Professor of Medicine and Pathology, University of Virginia School of Medicine, Unites States of America

Dr Rita Helfand, Centers for Disease Control and Prevention, United States of America

Dr Simon Jenkins, Research Fellow, University of Birmingham Project on the ethical challenges experienced by British military healthcare professionals in the Ebola region, United Kingdom

Dr Pretesh Kiran, Assistant Professor, Community Health; Convener, Disaster Management Unit, St Johns National Academy of Health Sciences, India

Dr Markus Kirchner, Department for Infectious Disease Epidemiology, Robert Koch Institute, Germany

Dr Katherine Littler, Senior Policy Adviser, Wellcome Trust, United Kingdom

Professor Samuel McConkey, Head, International Health and Tropical Medicine, Royal College of Surgeons, Ireland

Dr Farhat Moazam, Founding Chairperson, Center of Biomedical Ethics and Culture, Sindh Institute of Urology and Transplantation, Pakistan

Dr Robert Nelson, Deputy Director and Senior Pediatric Ethicist, Office of Pediatric Therapeutics, Food and Drug Administration, United States of America

Professor Alistair Nichol, Consultant Anaesthetist, School of Medicine and Medical Sciences, and EU projects, University College Dublin, Ireland

Professor Lisa Schwartz, Arnold Johnson Chair in Health Care Ethics, Ethics in Health Care, McMaster University, Canada

Professor Michael Selgelid, Director, Centre for Human Bioethics, Monash University, Australia

Dr Kadri Simm, Associate Professor of Practical Philosophy, University of Tartu, Estonia

Dr Aissatou Touré, Head, Immunology Department, Institut Pasteur de Dakar and Member, National Ethics Committee, Senegal

Professor Ross Upshur, Canada Research Chair in Primary Care Research; Professor, Department of Family and Community Medicine and Dalla Lana School of Public Health, University of Toronto, Canada

Dr Maria Van Kerkhove, Centre for Global Health, Institut Pasteur, France

Dr Aminu Yakubu, Department of Health Planning and Research, Federal Ministry of Health, Nigeria

资源提供者

Professor Carl Coleman (Rapporteur), Professor of Law and Academic Director, Division of Online Learning, Seton Hall University, New Jersey, United States of America

世界卫生组织总部秘书处，瑞士日内瓦

Dr Vânia de la Fuente-Núñez, Technical Officer, Global Health Ethics, Department of Knowledge, Ethics and Research

Dr Andreas Reis, Technical Officer, Global Health Ethics, Department of Knowledge, Ethics and Research

Dr Abha Saxena, Coordinator, Global Health Ethics, Department of Knowledge, Ethics and Research

制定世界卫生组织伦理和流行病指南的会议，意大利普拉托，2015 年 11 月 22 日至 24 日

参加者

Dr Franklyn Prieto Alvarado, Universidad Nacional de Colombia, Colombia

Dr Annick Antierens, Médecins Sans Frontières, Switzerland

Professor Oumou Younoussa Bah-Sow, Ignace Deen National Hospital, Guinea

Dr Ruchi Baxi, The Ethox Centre, United Kingdom

Dr Ron Bayer, Mailman School of Public Health, United States of America

Dr Oscar Cabrera, Executive Director, O'Neill Institute for National and Global Health Law, Georgetown University Law Center, United States of America

Dr Philippe Calain, Senior Researcher, Research on Humanitarian Stakes and Practices, Médecins Sans Frontières, Switzerland

Dr Voo Teck Chuan, National Academy of Health Sciences, India

Professor Alice Desclaux, Institut de Recherche pour le Développement, Unité TRANSVIHMI, Centre Régional de Recherche et de Formation sur le VIH et les Maladies Associées, Hôpital de Fann, Sénégal

Dr Benedict Dossen, National Research Ethics Board, University of Liberia–Pacific Institute for Research and Evaluation, Africa Center Institutional Review Board, Liberia

Dr Sarah Edwards, Research Ethics and Governance, University College London, United Kingdom

Professor Amy F Fairchild, Mailman School of Public Health, United States of America Dr Eddy Foday, Ministry of Health and Sanitation, Sierra Leone

Professor Frederick G Hayden, Mailman School of Public Health, United States of America

Dr Amar Jesani, Yenepoya University, India

Ms Rebecca Johnson, Ebola survivor, Sierra Leone

Ms Robinah Kaitiritimba, Patient representative (Community representative, Makerere University Institutional Review Board; Uganda National Health Consumers' Organisation, Uganda

Dr Stephen Kennedy, Coordinator, Ebola Virus Disease Research, Incident Management System, Liberia

Dr Pretesh Kiran, National Academy of Health Sciences, India

Professor Mark Leys, Vrije Universiteit Brussel,Belgium

Dr Farhat Moazam, Founding Chairperson of Center of Biomedical Ethics and Culture, Sindh Institute of Urology and Transplantation, Pakistan

Dr Dónal O'Mathúna, Dublin City University, Ireland

Professor Mahmudur Rahman, Director, Institute of Epidemiology, Disease Control and Research; National Influenza Center, Ministry of Health and Family Welfare, Bangladesh

Professor Lisa Schwartz, Arnold Johnson Chair in Health Care Ethics, McMaster Ethics in Healthcare, McMaster University, Canada

Professor Michael Selgelid, Director, Centre for Human Bioethics, Monash University, Australia

Dr Aissatou Touré, Head, Immunology Unit, Institut Pasteur de Dakar, Senegal

Dr Maria Van Kerkhove, Centre for Global Health, Institut Pasteur, France

观察员

Dr Katherine Littler, Senior Policy Adviser, Policy Department, Wellcome Trust, United Kingdom

资源顾问

Professor Carl Coleman, Professor of Law and Academic Director, Division of Online Learning, Seton Hall University, New Jersey, United States of America

Dr Michele Loi (Rapporteur), Post-doctoral research fellow, ETH Zürich, Switzerland

Dr Diego Silva, Assistant Professor, Faculty of Health Sciences, Simon Fraser University, Canada

世界卫生组织总部秘书处，瑞士日内瓦

Dr Pierre Formenty, Scientist, Control of Epidemic Diseases, Department of Pandemic and Epidemic Diseases

Dr Vânia de la Fuente-Núñez, Technical Officer, Global Health Ethics, Department of Knowledge, Ethics and Research

Dr Andreas Reis, Technical Officer Global Health Ethics, Department of Knowledge, Ethics and Research

Dr Abha Saxena, Coordinator, Global Health Ethics, Department of Knowledge, Ethics and Research

附件 3：译者的话

2014 年 8 月，埃博拉病毒疫情被宣布为国际关注的突发公共卫生事件。大家看到，传染病暴发期间的紧急决策，通常是处在科学的不确定性、社会和机构混乱，以及恐惧和不信任的总体气氛背景之下，面临诸如有效的疫情监控、及时真实透明的信息公开、社区参与、污名化和歧视、稀缺资源分配、限制行动自由、管理医疗干预、开展科学研究，以及一线工作人员的权利和义务等等问题。世界卫生组织认识到，这些伦理问题也普遍存在于其他全球传染病暴发的管理实践之中，于是在 2016 年发布了《传染病暴发伦理问题管理指南》。

时值我国众志成城抗击新冠肺炎疫情的关键阶段，世界卫生组织的这个指南从伦理问题的角度，对疫情防控期间的公共政策和社会治理都提出了许多有益的原则和建议。他山之石，可以攻玉，这些宝贵的经验都是在无数人痛苦甚至牺牲的基础上获得的，不仅对当下疫情防控的具体实践具有借鉴意义，也对从治理能力和治理体系方面补短板、强弱项，完善我国重大疫情防控体制机制，健全国家公共卫生应急管理体系提供了参考。我们突击翻译了这个指南，衷心希望能够对正在奋力抗击新冠肺炎疫情的人们有所启发和帮助。

在此，我们要特别感谢世界卫生组织，得知我们的意愿后，按照紧急情况第一时间授权我们翻译出版；感谢张奇先生、Aditi Bana 和 Carla ABOU MRAD 给予的大力支持和指导帮助！

熊宁宁

2020 年 2 月 18 日

Guidance for Managing Ethical Issues in Infectious Disease Outbreaks

World Health Organization 2016

Table of Contents

Foreword

Infectious disease outbreaks are periods of great uncertainty. Events unfold, resources and capacities that are often limited are stretched yet further, and decisions for a public health response must be made quickly, even though the evidence for decision-making may be scant. In such a situation, public health officials, policy-makers, funders, researchers, field epidemiologists, first responders, national ethics boards, health-care workers, and public health practitioners need a moral compass to guide them in their decision-making .

Bioethics puts people at the heart of the problem, emphasizes the principles that should guide health systems, and provides the moral rationale for making choices, particularly in a crisis .

I therefore welcome the development of the *Guidance for managing ethical issues in infectious disease outbreaks,* which will be key to embedding ethics within the integrated global alert and response system for epidemics and other public health emergencies. The publication will also support and strengthen the implementation and uptake of policies and programmes in this context .

Research is an integral part of the public health response – not only to learn about the current epidemic but also to build an evidence base for future epidemics. Research during an epidemic ranges from epidemiological and socio-behavioral to clinical trials and toxicity studies, all of which are crucial. I am pleased to see that the guidance touches upon this important area with advice, not only on research and emergency use of unproven interventions, but also on rapid data sharing see: http://www.who.int/ihr/procedures/SPG_data_sharing.pdf?ua=1.

The importance given to communication during an infectious disease outbreak can make or break public health efforts, and WHO takes this very seriously. This document outlines the ethical principles that should guide communication planning and implementation at every level from frontline workers to policy-makers .

The guidance represents the work of an international group of stakeholders and experts, including public health practitioners in charge of response management at the local, national and international level; nongovernmental organization representatives; directors of funding agencies; chairs of ethics committees; heads of research laboratories; representatives of national regulatory agencies; patient representatives; and experts in public health ethics, bioethics, human rights, anthropology, and epidemiology. I am grateful for their support and input .

Dr Marie-Paule Kieny

Assistant Director-General

Health Systems and Innovation

Acknowledgements

The Guidance document was produced under the overall direction of Abha Saxena, Coordinator of the Global Health Ethics team, supported by Andreas Reis and Maria Magdalena Guraiib .

WHO is grateful to Carl Coleman for his role as lead writer, his analysis and synthesis of existing guidance documents, and his incorporation of comments generated during preparatory meetings and the broader peer review process.

Appreciation is extended to the many individuals and organizations who provided comments on drafts of the guidance document, including: Alice Desclaux, Institut de Recherche pour le Développement, France; Aminu Yakubu, Federal Ministry of Health, Nigeria; Annick Antierens, Médecins Sans Frontières, Belgium; Bagher Larijani, Endocrinology and Metabolism Research Center, Iran (Islamic Republic of); Brad Freeman, Washington University School of Medicine, USA; Catherine Hankins, Amsterdam Institute for Global Health and Development, Netherlands; Cheryl Macpherson, Bioethics Department, St. George's University School of Medicine, Grenada; Claude Vergès, Universidad de Panamá, Panama; Drue H Barrett, Nicole J Cohen, and Rita F Helfand, Centers for Disease Control and Prevention, USA; Dirceu Greco, Federal University of Minas Gerais, Brazil; Edward Foday, Ministry of Health and Sanitation, Sierra Leone; Emilie Alirol, Geneva University Hospitals, Switzerland; Heather Draper, University of Birmingham, United Kingdom; Kenneth Goodman, Miller School of Medicine, University of Miami, USA; Morenike Oluwatoyin Ukpong, Obafemi Awolowo University, Nigeria; Paul Bouvier, International Committee of the Red Cross, Switzerland; Ruth Macklin, Albert Einstein College of Medicine, USA; Voo Tech Chuan, Centre for Biomedical Ethics, National University of Singapore, Singapore.

The advice, comments and guidance of the following entities are also gratefully acknowledged: COST Action IS 1201: Disaster Bioethics (in particular Dónal O'Mathúna, Dublin City University, Ireland; the staff of the Nuffield Council on Bioethics, United Kingdom (in particular Hugh Whittall); Johns Hopkins Berman Institute of Bioethics, USA (in particular Nancy Kass and Jeffrey Kahn); the International Severe Acute Respiratory and Emerging Infection Consortium, United Kingdom and its members (in particular Alistair Nichol, Irish Critical Care–Clinical Research Core, University College Dublin, Ireland, and Raul Pardinaz-Solis, Centre for Tropical Medicine and Global Health, University of Oxford, United Kingdom); and the Secretariat of the National Committee of Bioethics, King Abdulaziz City for Science and Technology, Kingdom of Saudi Arabia.

WHO appreciates the collaboration of the Chairperson (Christiane Woopen, then Chair of the German Ethics Council) and members of the Steering Committee of the Global Summit of National Ethics/Bioethics Committees, who provided the opportunity to present an earlier draft of the Guidance to representatives of 83 national ethics committees at the Summit in Berlin in March 2016. Their review and comments have been incorporated into this document.

The document also benefited from the review of the Global Network of WHO Collaborating Centers on Bioethics. Special thanks go to Ronald Bayer, the outgoing Chair of this network, and Amy Fairchild, Chair of the Guideline Development Group for the ethics of public health surveillance (both from Mailman School of Public Health, Columbia University, USA), and to the incoming Chair of the network, Michael Selgelid, Center for Human Bioethics, Monash University, Australia. The critical review by these individuals ensured that the guidance document was consistent with other ongoing projects.

Many frontline responders and WHO staff members who are routinely challenged during epidemic outbreaks provided valuable contributions based on their personal experiences; the document is much richer in its content as a result. The WHO Research Ethics Committee and the Public Health Ethics Consultative Group provided valuable inputs, drawing especially on their review of research and public health projects undertaken during the Ebola and Zika outbreaks.

WHO gratefully acknowledges the input of Ross Upshur, University of Toronto, Canada (first chair of the Ethics Working Group), and the subsequent co-chairs Lisa Schwartz, McMaster University, Canada, and Aissatou Touré, Institut Pasteur de Dakar, Senegal. Both co-chairs spent countless hours with the Secretariat and the lead writer to review thoughtfully the many comments received and to give final shape to the document. Philippe Calain, Médecins Sans Frontières, Switzerland, Chair of the Ethics Panel and a member of various ethics working groups, continuously challenged the WHO Secretariat to look beyond science to the people affected by the outbreaks, their cultures and their societies.

The guidance document specifically benefited from reviews of the following WHO staff: Juliet Bedford, Carla Saenz Bresciani, Ian Clarke, Rudi J J M Coninx, Pierre Formenty, Gaya Manori Gamhewage, Theo Grace, Paul Gully, Brooke Ronald Johnson JR, Annette Kuesel, Anaïs Legand, Ahmed Mohamed Amin Mandil, Bernadette Murgue, Tim Nguyen, Asiya Ismail Odugleh-Kolev, Martin Matthew Okechukwu Ota, Bruce Jay Plotkin, Annie Portela, Marie-Pierre Preziosi, Manju Rani, Nigel Campbell Rollins, Cathy Roth, Manisha Shridhar, Rajesh Sreedharan, David Wood, and Yousef Elbes.

A special thanks to Vânia de la Fuente Núñez, who was responsible for managing the Ethics Working Group; and Michele Loi who coordinated the whole process. Former interns of the Global Health Ethics team Patrick Hummel (University of St Andrews, United Kingdom) and Corinna Klingler (University of Munich, Germany) deserve a special mention for undertaking a scoping review in relation to pregnancy and infectious diseases, which informed the development of guidance in this area.

The guidance document would not have been possible without the generous support of the Wellcome Trust. The kind support of the following partners is also very gratefully acknowledged: 3U Global Health Partnership; Canadian Institutes of Health Research; Dublin City University; European Union Cooperation in Science and Technology; Monash University; University of Miami Miller School of Medicine Institute for Bioethics and Health Policy.

Introduction

This guidance grew out of concern at the World Health Organization (WHO) about ethical issues raised by the Ebola outbreak in West Africa in 2014–2016. The WHO Global Health Ethics Unit's response to Ebola began in August 2014, immediately after it was declared a "public health emergency of international concern" pursuant to the *International Health Regulations (2005)* (IHR).[1] That declaration led to the formation of an Ethics Panel, and later an Ethics Working Group, which was charged with developing ethics guidance on issues and concerns as they arose in the course of the epidemic. It became increasingly apparent that the ethical issues raised by Ebola mirrored concerns that had arisen in other global infectious disease outbreaks, including severe acute respiratory syndrome (SARS), pandemic influenza, and multidrug-resistant tuberculosis. However, while WHO has issued ethical guidance on some of these outbreaks,[2,3,4,5] prior guidance has only focused on the specific pathogen in isolation. The purpose of this document is to look beyond issues specific to particular epidemic pathogens and instead focus on the cross-cutting ethical issues that apply to infectious disease outbreaks generally. In addition to setting forth general principles, it examines how these principles can be adapted to different epidemiological and social circumstances .

While many of the ethical issues that arise in infectious disease outbreaks are the same as those that arise in other areas of public health, the context of an outbreak has particular complexities . Decisions during an outbreak need to be made on an urgent basis, often in the context of scientific uncertainty, social and institutional disruption, and an overall climate of fear and distrust. Invariably, the countries most affected by outbreaks have limited resources, underdeveloped legal and regulatory structures, and health systems that lack the resilience to deal with crisis situations. Countries that experience natural disasters and armed conflicts are particularly at risk, as these circumstances simultaneously increase the risk of infectious disease outbreaks while decreasing needed resources and access to health care. Moreover, infectious disease outbreaks can generate or exacerbate social crises that can weaken already fragile health systems. Within such contexts, it is not possible to satisfy all urgent needs simultaneously, forcing decision-makers to weigh and prioritize potentially competing ethical values. Time pressures and resource constraints may force action without the thorough deliberation, inclusiveness and transparency that a robust ethical decision-making process demands .

This guidance document on ethical issues that arise specifically in the context of infectious disease outbreaks aims to complement existing guidance on ethics in public health. It should therefore be read in conjunction with more general guidance on issues such as public health surveillance, research with human participants, and addressing the needs of vulnerable populations.

Setting up decision-making systems and procedures in advance is the best way to ensure that ethically appropriate decisions will be made if an outbreak occurs. Countries, health-care institutions, international organizations and others involved in epidemic response efforts are encouraged to develop practical strategies and tools to apply the principles in this guidance document to their specific settings, taking into account local social, cultural, and political contexts. WHO is committed to providing countries with technical assistance in support of these efforts .

Relevant ethical principles

Ethics involves judgements about "the way we ought to live our lives, including our actions, intentions, and our habitual behaviour."[3] The process of ethical analysis involves identifying relevant principles, applying them to a particular situation, and making judgements about how to weigh competing principles when it is not possible to satisfy them all. This guidance document draws on a variety of ethical principles, which are grouped below into seven general categories. These categories are presented merely for the convenience of the reader; other ways of grouping them are equally legitimate .

Justice — As used in this document, justice, or fairness, encompasses two different concepts. The first is *equity*, which refers to fairness in the distribution of resources, opportunities and outcomes . Key elements of equity include treating like cases alike, avoiding discrimination and exploitation, and being sensitive to persons who are especially vulnerable to harm or injustice. The second aspect of justice is *procedural justice*, which refers to a fair process for making important decisions . Elements of procedural justice include due process (providing notice to interested persons and an opportunity to be heard), transparency (providing clear and accurate information about the basis for decisions and the process by which they are made), inclusiveness/community engagement (ensuring all relevant stakeholders are able to participate in decisions), accountability (allocating and enforcing responsibility for decisions), and oversight (ensuring appropriate mechanisms for monitoring and review) .

Beneficence — Beneficence refers to acts that are done for the benefit of others, such as efforts to relieve individuals' pain and suffering. In the public health context, the principle of beneficence underlies society's obligation to meet the basic needs of individuals and communities, particularly humanitarian needs such as nourishment, shelter, good health, and security .

Utility — The principle of utility states that actions are right insofar as they promote the well-being of individuals or communities. Efforts to maximize utility require consideration of proportionality (balancing the potential benefits of an activity against any risks of harm) and efficiency (achieving the greatest benefits at the lowest possible cost) .

Respect for persons — The term "respect for persons" refers to treating individuals in ways that are fitting to and informed by a recognition of our common humanity, dignity and inherent rights. A central aspect of respect for persons is respect for autonomy, which requires letting individuals make their own choices based on their values and preferences. Informed consent, a process in which a competent individual authorizes a course of action based on sufficient relevant information, without coercion or undue inducement, is one way to operationalize this concept. Where individuals lack decision-making capacity, it may be necessary for others to be charged with protecting their interests. Respect for persons also includes paying attention to values such as privacy and confidentiality, as well as social, religious and cultural beliefs and important relationships, including family bonds. Finally, respect for persons requires transparency and truth-telling in the context of carrying out public health and research activities .

Liberty — Liberty includes a broad range of social, religious and political freedoms, such as freedom of movement, freedom of peaceful assembly, and freedom of speech . Many aspects of liberty are protected as fundamental human rights .

Reciprocity — Reciprocity consists of making a "fitting and proportional return" for contributions that people have made.[6] Policies that encourage reciprocity can be an important means of promoting the principle of justice, as they can correct unfair disparities in the distribution of the benefits and burdens of epidemic response efforts .

Solidarity — Solidarity is a social relation in which a group, community, nation or, potentially, global community stands together.[7] The principle of solidarity justifies collective action in the face of common threats. It also supports efforts to overcome inequalities that undermine the welfare of minorities and groups that suffer from discrimination .

Practical applications

The application of ethical principles should be informed by evidence as far as it is available. For example, in determining whether a particular action contributes to utility, decision-makers should be guided by any available scientific evidence about the action's expected benefits and harms . The more intrusive the proposed action, the greater the need for robust evidence that what is being proposed is likely to achieve its desired aim. When specific evidence is not available, decisions should be based on reasoned, substantive arguments and informed by evidence from analogous situations, to the extent possible .

In balancing competing principles during infectious disease outbreaks, countries must respect their obligations under international human rights agreements. The *Siracusa Principles on the Limitation and Derogation Provisions in the International Covenant on Civil and Political Rights* (the "Siracusa Principles")[8] are a widely accepted framework for evaluating the appropriateness of limiting certain fundamental human rights in emergency situations. The Siracusa Principles provide that any restrictions on human rights must be carried out in accordance with the law and in pursuit of a legitimate objective of general interest. In addition, such restrictions must be strictly necessary and there must be no other, less intrusive means available to reach the same objective. Finally, any restrictions must be based on scientific evidence and not imposed in an arbitrary, unreasonable, or discriminatory manner . [10]

For both pragmatic and ethical reasons, maintaining the population's trust in epidemic response efforts is of fundamental importance. This is possible only if policy-makers and response workers act in a trustworthy manner by applying procedural principles fairly and consistently, being open to review based on new relevant information, and acting with the genuine input of affected communities.

In addition, a synchronized approach is indispensable to the success of any response effort. All members of the global community need to act in solidarity, since all countries share a common vulnerability to the threat of infectious disease.

How the Guidance was developed

Many individuals have helped shape this guidance document, directly or indirectly, starting with the Ethics Panel that was convened by the Director-General on 11 August 2014, and the ad-hoc ethics working groups that met in Geneva, Switzerland between August and October 2014 to provide guidance on the use of untested interventions during the Ebola outbreak in West Africa. Subsequently, in May 2015, a group of experts and stakeholders met in Dublin, Ireland to review existing ethical statements on infectious disease outbreaks and develop a methodology to create a more comprehensive document. To assist this process, an analysis and synthesis of all existing guidance documents relevant to ethical considerations in infectious disease outbreaks was prepared (Annex 1). Reflecting on lessons learnt from previous outbreaks, particularly the recent experiences with Ebola, participants emphasized the need for guidance that could be tailored to different epidemiological, social, and economic contexts. They also discussed the importance of focusing on broader questions of global health governance, community engagement, knowledge generation, and priority setting. Finally, participants emphasized the urgent need to develop concrete operational tools to help individuals involved in epidemic response efforts to incorporate ethical guidance into practical decision-making. The group met again in November 2015 in Prato, Italy to review an initial draft of the guidance and to hear from additional experts and stakeholders, including survivors of the recent Ebola outbreak. Following this meeting, a new draft was developed and circulated for international peer review. The experts that participated in these meetings to prepare the Guidelines are listed in Annex 2.

This document is organized around 14 specific guidelines, each of which addresses key aspects of epidemic planning and response. Each guideline is introduced by a series of questions that illustrate the scope of the ethical issues, followed by a more detailed discussion that articulates the rights and obligations of relevant stakeholders. It is hoped that this document will be useful to policy-makers, public health professionals, health-care providers, frontline responders, researchers, pharmaceutical and medical device companies, and other relevant entities involved in infectious disease outbreaks planning and response efforts in the public and private sectors.

Guidelines

1. Obligations of governments and the international community

Questions addressed:

- What are the obligations of governments to prevent and respond to infectious disease outbreaks?
- Why do countries' obligations to prevent and respond to infectious disease outbreaks extend beyond their own borders?
- What obligations do countries have to participate in global surveillance and preparedness efforts?
- What obligations do governments have to provide financial, technical, and scientific assistance to countries in need?

Governments can play a critical role in preventing and responding to infectious disease outbreaks by improving social and environmental conditions, ensuring well-functioning and accessible health systems, and engaging in public health surveillance and prevention activities. Together, these actions can substantially reduce the spread of diseases with epidemic potential. In addition, they help assure that an effective public health response will be possible if an epidemic occurs. Governments have an ethical obligation to ensure the long-term capacity of the systems necessary to carry out effective epidemic prevention and response efforts.

Countries have obligations not only to persons within their own borders but also to the broader international community. As the United Nations Committee on Economic, Social and Cultural Rights has recognized, "given that some diseases are easily transmissible beyond the frontiers of a State, the international community has a collective responsibility to address this problem. The economically developed States Parties have a special responsibility and interest to assist the poorer developing States in this regard."[9]

These obligations reflect the practical reality that infectious disease outbreaks do not respect national borders, and that an outbreak in one country can put the rest of the world at risk.

Countries' obligations to consider the needs of the international community do not arise solely in times of emergency. Instead, they require ongoing attention to ameliorate the social determinants of poor health that contribute to infectious disease outbreaks, including poverty, limited access to education, and inadequate systems of water and sanitation.

The following are key elements of the obligations of governments and the international community:

- ***Ensuring the sufficiency of national public health laws*** — As discussed later in this document, certain public health interventions that might be necessary during an infectious disease outbreak (e.g. restrictions on freedom of movement) depend on having a clear legal basis for government action, as well as a system in place to provide oversight and review. All countries should review their public health laws to ensure that they give the government sufficient authority to respond effectively to an epidemic while also providing individuals with appropriate human rights protections.

- ***Participating in global surveillance and preparedness efforts*** — All countries must carry out their responsibilities under the IHR to participate in global surveillance efforts in a truthful and transparent manner. This includes providing prompt notification of events that may constitute a public health emergency of international concern, regardless of any negative consequences that may be associated with notification, such as a possible reduction in trade or tourism. The obligation to provide prompt notification to the international community stems not only from the text of the IHR but also from the ethical principles of solidarity and reciprocity. In addition, countries should develop preparedness plans for infectious disease outbreaks and other potential disasters and provide guidance to relevant health-care facilities to implement the plans.

- ***Providing financial, technical, and scientific assistance*** — Countries that have the resources to provide foreign assistance should support global epidemic preparedness and response efforts, including research and development on diagnostics, therapeutics, and vaccines for pathogens with epidemic potential. This support should supplement ongoing efforts to build local public health capacities and strengthen primary health care systems in countries at greatest risk of harm from infectious disease outbreaks.

2. Involving the local community

> **Questions addressed:**
> - Why is community engagement a critical component of infectious disease outbreak response efforts?
> - What are the hallmarks of a community-centred approach to infectious disease outbreak response?
> - What should decision-makers do with input they receive during community engagement activities?
> - What is the media's role in infectious disease outbreak response efforts?

All aspects of infectious disease outbreak response efforts should be supported by early and ongoing engagement with the affected communities. In addition to being ethically important in its own right, community engagement is essential to establishing and maintaining trust and preserving social order.

Involving communities fully in infectious disease outbreak planning and response efforts requires attention to the following issues:

- *Inclusiveness* — All persons who could potentially be affected should have opportunities to make their voices heard in all stages of infectious disease outbreak planning and response, either directly or through legitimate representatives. Adequate communication platforms and tools should be put in place to facilitate public communication with health authorities.

- *Situations of particular vulnerability* — As discussed further in Guideline 3, special attention should be given to ensuring that persons who face heightened susceptibility to harm or injustice during infectious disease outbreaks are able to contribute to decisions about infectious disease outbreak planning and response. Public health officials should recognize that such persons might be distrustful of government and other institutions, and make special efforts to include them in community engagement plans.

- *Openness to diverse perspectives* — Communication efforts should be designed to facilitate a genuine two-way dialogue, rather than as merely a means to announce decisions that have already been made

Decision-makers should be prepared to recognize and debate alternative approaches and revise their decisions based on information they receive. Reaching out to the community early, and allowing for consideration of the interests of all people who will potentially be affected, can play an important role in building trust and empowering communities to be involved in a genuine dialogue.

• *Transparency* — The ethical principle of transparency requires that decision-makers publicly explain the basis for decisions in language that is linguistically and culturally appropriate. When decisions must be made in the face of uncertain information, the uncertainties should be explicitly acknowledged and conveyed to the public.

• *Accountability* — The public should know who is responsible for making Cholera outbreak in Sierra Leone and implementing decisions in relation to the outbreak response, and how they can challenge decisions they believe are inappropriate.

The media will play an important role in any infectious disease outbreak response effort. It is therefore important to ensure that the media has access to accurate and timely information about the disease and its management. Governments, nongovernmental organizations, and academic institutions should make efforts to support media training in relevant scientific concepts and techniques for communicating risk information without raising unnecessary alarm. Media training is important for public health sector employees who may interact with media covering public health issues. In turn, the media has a responsibility to provide accurate, factual, and balanced reporting. This is an important component of media ethics.

3. Situations of particular vulnerability

Questions addressed:

- Why are some individuals and groups considered particularly vulnerable during infectious disease outbreaks?

- How can vulnerability affect a person's ability to access services during infectious disease outbreaks?

- How can vulnerability affect a person's willingness and ability to share and receive information during an infectious disease outbreak?

- Why are stigmatization and discrimination particular risks during infectious disease outbreaks?

- In what ways might vulnerable persons suffer disproportionate burdens from infectious disease response efforts, or have a greater need for resources?

Some individuals and groups face heightened susceptibility to harm or injustice during infectious disease outbreaks. Policy-makers and epidemic responders should develop plans to address the needs of such individuals and groups in advance of an outbreak and, if an outbreak occurs, make reasonable efforts to ensure that these needs are actually met. Doing this requires ongoing attention to community engagement and the development of active social networks between community representatives and government actors.

Efforts to address the ways in which individuals and groups may be vulnerable should take into account the following:

- *Difficulty accessing services and resources* — Many of the characteristics that contribute to social vulnerability can make it difficult for individuals to access necessary services. For example, persons with physical disabilities may have mobility impairments that make travelling even short distances difficult or impossible. Other socially vulnerable persons may lack access to safe and reliable transportation or have caregiving responsibilities that make it difficult for them to leave their homes. In addition, vulnerable persons may lack access to necessary resources such as clean water or bednets to reduce the risk of contracting a mosquito-borne disease.

- *Need for effective alternative communication strategies* — Some types of vulnerability can impede an individual's ability to transmit or receive information. Communication barriers can stem from a wide range of factors including, but not limited to, illiteracy, unfamiliarity with the local or official language(s), vision or hearing impairments, social isolation, or lack of access to Internet and other communication services. These barriers make it difficult for individuals to receive necessary public health messages or to participate fully in community engagement activities. To overcome these barriers, messages should be delivered in multiple formats (e.g. radio, text messages, billboards, cartoons) as well as direct oral communication with key stakeholders. Health authorities should not assume that the public will search for information; instead, they should proactively reach out to the concerned population wherever they are.

- *Impact of stigmatization and discrimination* — Members of socially disadvantaged groups often face considerable stigma and discrimination, which can be exacerbated in public health emergencies characterized by fear and distrust. Those responsible for infectious disease outbreak response should ensure that all individuals are treated fairly and equitably regardless of their social status or perceived "worth" to society. They should also take measures to prevent stigmatization and social violence.

- *Disproportionate burdens of outbreak response measures* — Even when public health measures are designed with the best of intentions, they can inadvertently place a disproportionate burden on particular populations. For example, quarantine orders that require individuals to stay in their homes can have devastating consequences for persons who need to leave their homes to obtain basic necessities such as clean water or food. Similarly, social distancing measures such as school closures can place disproportionate burdens on children who depend on going to school to access regular meals, as well as on working parents who may have no one available to provide child care.

- *Greater need for resources* — Accommodating the needs of individuals whose situation makes them particularly vulnerable sometimes requires the use of additional resources. In some cases, additional resources are relatively minimal, such as when an interpreter is hired to make a community engagement forum accessible to members of a linguistic minority group. In other cases, they may be more substantial, such as when mobile health teams are assembled to dispatch vaccines and treatments to hard-to-reach rural areas. It is legitimate to take costs into consideration in determining whether a particular accommodation is warranted; indeed, the goal of maximizing utility demands that such assessments be made. However, despite the importance of conserving limited resources, the ethical principle of equity may sometimes justify providing greater resources to persons who have greater needs.

- *Heightened risk of violence* — Infectious disease outbreaks can exacerbate social unrest, increase criminality, and induce violent behaviour, especially against vulnerable groups such as minority populations or migrants. In addition, public health measures such as home isolation, quarantine, or closure of schools and work facilities can induce violence, particularly against women and children. Officials involved in outbreak planning and response efforts should be prepared for the possibility that specific populations may be targeted as being the cause of the outbreak or provoking transmission; strategies should be proactively designed to protect members of such groups from a heightened risk of violence.

4. Allocating scarce resources

Questions addressed:

• What type of resource allocation decisions might need to be made during infectious disease outbreaks?

• How do the principles of utility and equity apply to decisions about allocating scarce resources during infectious disease outbreaks?

• How does the principle of reciprocity apply to decisions about allocating scarce resources during infectious disease outbreaks?

• What procedural considerations apply to decisions about resource allocation during infectious disease outbreaks?

• What obligations do health-care providers have towards persons who are not able to access life-saving resources during infectious disease outbreaks?

Infectious disease outbreaks can quickly overwhelm the capacities of governments and health-care systems, requiring them to make difficult decisions about the allocation of limited resources. Some of these decisions may arise in the context of allocating medical interventions, such as hospital beds, medications, and medical equipment. Others may relate to broader questions about how public health resources should be utilized. For example, how should limited resources be allocated between activities such as surveillance, health promotion, and community engagement? Should human resources be devoted to contact tracing at the possible expense of patient management? Should limited funds be spent improving water and sanitation facilities or building quarantine facilities?

Infectious disease outbreaks also compete with other important public health issues for attention and resources. For example, one of the consequences of the Ebola outbreak was a reduction in access to general health-care services due to a combination of a greater number of patients and the sickness and death of health-care workers. As a result, deaths from tuberculosis, human immunodeficiency virus (HIV), and malaria increased dramatically during this period.[10]

Governments, health-care facilities, and others involved in response efforts should prepare for such situations by developing guidelines on the allocation of scarce resources in outbreak situations. Such guidelines should be developed through an open and transparent process involving broad stakeholder input and, to the extent possible, should be incorporated into formal written documents that establish clear priorities and procedures. Those involved in developing these guidelines should be guided by the following considerations:

- *Balancing considerations of utility and equity* — Resource allocation decisions should be guided by the ethical principles of utility and equity. The principle of utility requires allocating resources to maximize benefits and minimize burdens, while the principle of equity requires attention to the fair distribution of benefits and burdens. In some cases, an equal distribution of benefits and burdens may be considered fair, but in others, it may be fairer to give preference to groups that are worse off, such as the poor, the sick, or the vulnerable. It is not always be possible to achieve fully both utility and equity. For example, establishing treatment centres in large urban settings promotes the value of utility because it makes it possible to treat a large number of people with relatively few resources. However, such an approach may be in tension with the principle of equity if it means that fewer resources will be directed to isolated communities in remote rural areas. There is no single correct way to resolve potential tensions between utility and equity; what is important is that decisions are made through an inclusive and transparent process that takes into account local circumstances.

- *Defining utility on the basis of health-related considerations* — In order to apply the ethical principle of utility, it is first necessary to identify the type of outcomes that will be counted as improvements to welfare. In general, the focus should be on the health-related benefits of allocation mechanisms, whether defined in terms of the total number of lives saved, the total number of life years saved, or the total number of quality-adjusted life years saved. For this reason, while it might be ethical to prioritize persons who are essential to manage an outbreak, it is not appropriate to prioritize persons based on social value considerations unrelated to carrying out critical services necessary for society.

- *Paying attention to the needs of vulnerable populations* — In applying the ethical principle of equity, special attention should be given to individuals and groups that are the most vulnerable to discrimination, stigmatization, or isolation, as discussed in Guideline[3]. Particular consideration must be given to individuals who are confined in institutional settings, where they are highly dependent on others and potentially exposed to much higher risks of infection than persons living in the community.

- *Fulfilling reciprocity-based obligations to those who contribute to infectious disease outbreak response efforts* — The ethical principle of reciprocity implies that society should support persons who face a disproportionate burden or risk in protecting the public good. This principle justifies giving priority access to scarce resources to persons who assume risks to their own health or life to contribute to outbreak response efforts.

- *Providing supportive and palliative care to persons unable to access lifesaving resources* — Even when it is not possible to provide life-saving medical resources to all who could benefit from them, efforts should be made to ensure that no patients are abandoned. One way to do this is to ensure that adequate resources are directed to providing supportive and palliative care.

The application of allocation principles should take into account the following considerations:

- **Consistent application** — Allocation principles should be applied in a consistent manner, both within individual institutions and, to the extent possible, across geographic areas. Decision-making tools should be developed to ensure that like cases are treated alike, and that no person receives better or worse treatment due to his or her social status or other factors not explicitly recognized in the allocation plan. Efforts should be made to avoid unintended systemic discrimination in the choice or application of allocation methods.

- **Resolution of disputes** — Mechanisms should be developed to resolve disagreements about the application of allocation principles; these mechanisms should be designed to ensure that anyone who believes that allocation principles have been applied inappropriately has access to impartial and accountable review processes, and has the opportunity to be heard.

- **Avoiding corruption** — Corruption in the health-care sector may be exacerbated during infectious disease outbreaks if large numbers of individuals are competing for access to limited resources. Efforts should be made to ensure that persons involved in the application of allocation systems do not accept or give bribes or engage in other corrupt activities.

- **Separation of responsibilities** — To the extent possible, the interpretation of allocation principles should not be entrusted to clinicians who have pre-existing professional relationships that create an ethical obligation to advocate for the interests of specific patients or groups. Instead, decisions should be made by appropriately qualified clinicians who have no personal or professional reasons to advocate for one patient or group over another.

5. Public health surveillance

Questions addressed:
- What role does surveillance play in infectious disease outbreak response efforts?
- Should surveillance activities be subject to ethical review?
- What obligations do entities conducting surveillance activities have to protect the confidentiality of information collected?
- Are there any circumstances under which individuals should be asked for consent to, or given the opportunity to opt out of, surveillance activities?
- What obligations do those conducting surveillance activities have to disclose information they collect to the affected individuals and communities?

Systematic observation and data collection are essential components of emergency response measures, both to guide the management of the current outbreak and to help prevent and respond to outbreaks in the future. Even if these activities are not characterized as research for regulatory purposes, an ethical analysis should be undertaken to ensure that personal information is protected from physical, legal, psychological, and other harm. Countries should consider organizing systems for ethical oversight of public health activities, commensurate with the activity objectives, methods, risks and benefits, as well as the extent to which the activity involves individuals or groups whose situation may make them vulnerable. Regardless of whether such systems are adopted, ethical analysis of public health activities should be consistent with accepted norms of public health ethics and conducted by individuals or entities that can be held accountable for their decisions.

Ensuring high-quality, ethically appropriate surveillance is complicated by at least two factors. First, the law surrounding surveillance across jurisdictions may be unnecessarily complex or inconsistent. Second, surveillance activities will occur across jurisdictions with varying levels of resources, thus placing strains on the quality and reliability of the data. These issues are likely to be exacerbated during an infectious disease outbreak, creating an urgent need for careful planning and international collaboration. Specific issues that should be addressed include the following:

- ***Protecting the confidentiality of personal information*** — The unauthorized disclosure of personal information collected during an infectious disease outbreak (including name, address, diagnosis, family history, etc.) can expose individuals to significant risk. Countries should ensure that adequate protection exists against these risks, including laws that safeguard the confidentiality of information generated through surveillance activities, and that strictly limit the circumstances in which such information may be used or disclosed for purposes different from those for which it was initially collected. Use and sharing of non-aggregated surveillance data for research purposes must have the approval of a properly constituted and trained research ethics committee.

- ***Assessing the importance of universal participation*** — Public health surveillance is typically conducted on a mandatory basis, without the possibility of individual refusal. Collecting surveillance information on a mandatory basis is ethically appropriate on the grounds of public interest if an accountable governmental authority has determined that universal participation is necessary to achieve compelling public health objectives. However, it should not be assumed that surveillance activities must always be carried out on a mandatory basis. Entities responsible for designing and approving surveillance programmes should consider the appropriateness of allowing individuals to opt out of particular surveillance activities, taking into account the nature and degree of individual risks involved and the extent to which allowing opt-outs would undermine the activity's public health goals

- ***Disclosing information to individuals and communities*** — Regardless of whether individuals are given the choice to opt out of surveillance activities, the process of surveillance should be conducted on a transparent basis. At a minimum, individuals and communities should be aware of the type of information that will be gathered about them, the purposes for which this information will be used, and any circumstances under which the information collected may be shared with third parties. In addition, information about the outcome of the surveillance activity should be made available as soon as reasonably possible. Careful attention should be given to the manner in which this information is communicated, in order to minimize the risk that subjects of surveillance may face stigmatization or discrimination

6. Restrictions on freedom of movement

> **Questions addressed:**
>
> • Under what circumstances is it legitimate to restrict an individual's freedom of movement during an infectious disease outbreak?
>
> • What living conditions should be assured for individuals whose freedom of movement has been restricted?
>
> • What other obligations are owed to individuals whose freedom of movement has been restricted?
>
> • What procedural protections must be established to ensure that restrictions on freedom of movement are carried out appropriately?
>
> • What are the obligations of policy-makers and public health officials to inform the public about restrictions on freedom of movement?

Restrictions on freedom of movement include isolation, quarantine, travel advisories or restrictions, and communitybased measures to reduce contact between people (e.g. closing schools or prohibiting large gatherings). These measures can often play an important role in controlling infectious disease outbreaks, and in these circumstances, their use is justified by the ethical value of protecting community wellbeing. However, the effectiveness of these measures should not be assumed; in fact, under some epidemiological circumstances, they may contribute little or nothing to outbreak control efforts, and may even be counterproductive if they engender a backlash that leads to resistance to other control measures. Moreover, all such measures impose a significant burden on individuals and communities, including direct limitations of fundamental human rights, particularly the rights to freedom of movement and peaceful assembly.

In light of these considerations, no restrictions on freedom of movement should be implemented without careful attention to the following considerations:

• *Justifiable basis for imposing restrictions* — Decisions to impose restrictions on freedom of movement should be grounded on the best available evidence about the outbreak pathogen, as determined in consultation with national and international public health officials. No such interventions should be implemented unless there is a reasonable basis to expect they will significantly reduce disease transmission. The rationale for relying on these measures should be made explicit, and the appropriateness of any restrictions should be continuously re-evaluated in light of emerging scientific information about the outbreak. If the original rationale for imposing a restriction no longer applies, the restriction should be lifted without delay.

• *Least restrictive means* — Any restrictions on freedom of movement should be designed and implemented in a manner that imposes the fewest constraints reasonably possible. Greater restrictions should be imposed only when there are strong grounds to believe that less restrictive measures are unlikely to achieve important public health goals. For example, requests for voluntary cooperation are generally preferable to public health mandates enforced by law or military authorities. Similarly, home-based quarantine should be considered before confining individuals in institutions. While isolation in a properly equipped healthcare facility is usually recommended for individuals who are already symptomatic, especially for diseases with a high potential for contagiousness, home-based isolation may sometimes be appropriate, provided that adequate medical and logistical support can be organized and family attendants are willing and able to act under the oversight of trained public health staff. This is particularly true if the caseload overwhelms facility capacity.

• *Costs* — In some cases, a less restrictive alternative may involve greater costs. This does not, in itself, justify more restrictive approaches. However, costs and other practical constraints (e.g logistics, distance, available workforce) may legitimately be taken into account to determine whether a less restrictive alternative is feasible under the circumstances, particularly in settings with severe resource constraints.

• *Ensuring humane conditions* — Any restrictions on freedom of movement, particularly those that are not voluntary, should be backed up with sufficient resources to ensure that those subject to the restrictions do not experience undue burdens. For example, individuals whose mobility is restricted (whether through confinement at home or in institutional settings) should be ensured access to food, drinking water, sanitary facilities, shelter, clothing, and medical care. It is also important to ensure that individuals have adequate physical space, opportunities to engage in activities, and the means to communicate with their loved ones and the outside world. Fulfilling these needs is essential to respect individual dignity and address the significant psychosocial burden of confinement on individuals and their loved ones. Mechanisms should be put in place to minimize the risk of violence (including sexual assault) and local disease transmission, especially when individuals are confined in institutional settings or when communities are under mass quarantine. At a minimum, persons who are quarantined because they have been exposed to the pathogen responsible for the outbreak should not be put at heightened risk of infection because of the manner in which they are confined. (Decisions on the circumstances and conditions of confinement should consider the heightened needs of vulnerable populations, as discussed in Guideline 3.)

- *Addressing financial and social consequences* — Even short-term restrictions on freedom of movement can have significant — and possibly devastating —financial and social consequences for individuals, their families, and their communities. Countries should provide assistance to households that suffer financial losses as a result of inability to conduct business, loss of a job, damage to crops, or other consequences of restrictions on freedom of movement. In some cases, this support may need to continue for a period following the end of confinement. In addition, efforts should be made to support the social and professional reintegration of individuals for whom confinement is no longer necessary, including measures to reduce stigmatization and discrimination.

- *Due process protections* — Mechanisms should be in place to allow individuals whose liberty has been restricted to challenge the appropriateness of those restrictions, the way they are enforced, and the conditions under which the restrictions are carried out. If it is not feasible to provide full due process protection before the restrictions are implemented in an emergency scenario, mechanisms for review and appeal should be made available without excessive delay. All persons involved in decisions to restrict individuals' freedom of movement should be accountable for any abuses of authority.

- *Equitable application* — Restrictions on freedom of movement should be applied in the same manner to all persons posing a comparable public health risk. Thus, individuals should not be subject to greater or lesser restrictions for reasons unrelated to the risks they may pose to others, including membership in any disfavoured or favoured social group or class (for example, groups defined by gender, ethnicity, or religion). In addition, policymakers should seek to ensure that restrictions are not applied in a manner that imposes a disproportionate burden on vulnerable segments of society.

- *Communication and transparency* — Policy-makers and public health officials should engage communities in a dialogue about any restrictions on freedom of movement and solicit community members' views on how restrictions can be carried out with the least possible burden. They should also provide regular updates on the implementation of such measures, both to the public at large and to those whose movement has been restricted. Communication strategies should be designed to avoid the stigmatization of individuals whose liberty has been restricted and to protect their privacy and confidentiality, particularly in the media.

7. Obligations related to medical interventions for the diagnosis, treatment, and prevention of infectious disease

> **Questions addressed:**
>
> • What quality and safety standards should govern the administration of medical interventions offered during infectious disease outbreaks?
>
> • What rights do patients (or their authorized proxy decision-makers) have to receive information about the risks and benefits of, and alternatives to, medical interventions during infectious disease outbreaks?
>
> • Under what circumstances, if any, might it be appropriate to override an individual's refusal of diagnostic, therapeutic, or preventive measures during an infectious disease outbreak?
>
> • What procedural safeguards should be provided before overriding an individual's refusal of diagnostic, therapeutic, or preventive measures during an infectious disease outbreak?

Any medical intervention for the diagnosis, treatment, or prevention of infectious disease should be provided in accord with professional medical standards, under conditions designed to ensure the highest attainable level of patient safety. Countries, with the support of international experts, should establish the minimum standards to be applied in the care and treatment of patients affected by an outbreak. These standards should apply not only to health-care institutions but also to home-based care, community activities (including health education sessions), and environmental decontamination efforts or the management of dead bodies.

Individuals offered medical interventions for the diagnosis, treatment, or prevention of an infectious pathogen should be informed about the risks, benefits, and alternatives, just as they would be for other significant medical interventions. The presumption should be that the final decision about which medical interventions to accept, if any, belongs to the patient. For patients who lack the legal capacity to make healthcare decisions for themselves, decisions should generally be made by appropriately authorized proxy decision-makers, with efforts made to solicit the patient's assent whenever possible.

Health-care providers should recognize that, in some situations, the refusal of diagnostic, therapeutic, or preventive measures might be a choice that is rational from the perspective of a mentally competent individual. If an individual is unwilling to accept an intervention, providers should engage the patient in an open and respectful dialogue, paying careful attention to the patient's concerns, perceptions, and situational needs.

In exceptional situations, there may be legitimate reasons to override an individual's refusal of a diagnostic, therapeutic, or preventive measure that has proven to be safe and effective and is part of the accepted medical standard of care. Decisions on whether to override a refusal should be grounded in the following considerations:

- *Public health necessity of the proposed intervention* — A mentally competent individual's refusal of diagnostic, therapeutic, or preventive measures should only be overridden when there is substantial reason to believe that accepting the refusal would pose significant risks to public health, that the intervention is likely to ameliorate those risks, and that no other measures to protect public health — including isolating the patient — are feasible under the circumstances.

- *Existence of medical contraindications to the proposed intervention* — Some interventions that may pose low risks for the majority of the population can pose heightened risks for individuals with particular medical conditions. Individuals should not be forced to undergo interventions that would expose them to significant risks in light of their personal medical circumstances.

- *Feasibility of providing interventions to an unwilling patient* — In some cases, it may be impossible to provide an intervention to an individual who is unwilling to be an active participant in the process. For example, standard treatment for tuberculosis requires the patient to take medication on a regular basis for several months. Without the patient's cooperation, it is unrealistic to expect that such a lengthy treatment regimen could successfully be completed. In such circumstances, the only realistic way to protect public health may be to isolate the patient until he or she is no longer infectious, assuming it is feasible to do so in a humane manner.

- *Impact on community trust* — Overriding individuals' refusal of diagnostic, therapeutic, or preventive measures can backfire if it leads members of the community to become distrustful of health-care providers or the public health system. Benefits from imposing unwanted interventions should be balanced against possible harms caused by undermining trust in the health-care system.

Objections to diagnostic, therapeutic, or preventive measures should not be overridden without giving the individual notice and an opportunity to raise his or her objections before an impartial decision maker, such as a court, interdisciplinary review panel, or other entity not involved in the initial decision. The burden should be on the proposer of the intervention to show that the expected public health benefits justify overriding the individual's choice. The process for resolving objections should be conducted in an open and transparent manner, consistent with the principles discussed in Guideline 2.

8. Research during infectious disease outbreaks

Questions addressed:

• What is the appropriate role of research during an infectious disease outbreak?

• How might the circumstances surrounding infectious disease outbreaks affect the ethical review of research proposals?

• How might the circumstances surrounding infectious disease outbreaks affect the process of informed consent to research?

• What methodological designs are appropriate for research conducted during infectious disease outbreaks?

• How should research be integrated into broader outbreak response efforts?

During an infectious disease outbreak there is a moral obligation to learn as much as possible as quickly as possible, in order to inform the ongoing public health response, and to allow for proper scientific evaluation of new interventions being tested. Such an approach will also improve preparedness for similar future outbreaks. Carrying out this obligation requires carefully designed and ethically conducted scientific research. In addition to clinical trials evaluating diagnostics, treatments or preventive measures such as vaccines, other types of research — including epidemiological, social science, and implementation studies — can play a critical role in reducing morbidity and mortality and addressing the social and economic consequences caused by the outbreak.

Research conducted during an infectious disease outbreak should be designed and implemented in conjunction with other public health interventions. Under no circumstances should research compromise the public health response to an outbreak or the provision of appropriate clinical care. All clinical trials must be prospectively registered in an appropriate clinical trial registry.

As in non-outbreak situations, it is essential to ensure that studies are scientifically valid and add social value; that risks are reasonable in relation to anticipated benefits; that participants are selected fairly and participate voluntarily (in most situations following an explicit process of informed consent); that participants' rights and well-being are sufficiently protected; and that studies undergo an adequate process of independent review. These internationally accepted norms and standards stem from the basic ethical principles of beneficence, respect for persons, and justice. They apply to all fields of research involving human beings, whether biomedical, epidemiological, public health or social science studies, and are explained in detail in numerous international ethics guidelines,[11,12,13,14,15] all of which apply with full force in outbreak situations. All actors in research, including researchers, research institutions, research ethics committees, national regulators, international organizations, and commercial sponsors, have an obligation to ensure that these principles are upheld in outbreak situations. Doing this requires attention to the following considerations:

- *Role of local research institutions* — When local researchers are available, they should be involved in the design, implementation, analysis, reporting and publication of outbreak-related research. Local researchers can help ensure that studies adequately respond to local realities and needs and that they can be implemented effectively without jeopardizing the emergency response. Involving local researchers in international research collaborations also contributes to building longterm research capacity in affected countries and promoting the value of international equity in science.

- *Addressing limitations in local research ethics review and scientific capacity* — Countries' capacity to engage in local research ethics review may be limited during outbreaks because of time constraints, lack of expertise, diversion of resources to outbreak response efforts, or pressure from public health authorities that undermines reviewers' independence. International and nongovernmental organizations should assist local research ethics committees to overcome these challenges by, for example, sponsoring collaborative reviews involving representatives from multiple countries supplemented by external experts.

- *Providing ethics review in timesensitive circumstances* — The need for immediate action to contain an infectious disease outbreak may make it impossible to adhere to the usual timeframes for research ethics review. National research governance systems and the international community should anticipate this problem by developing mechanisms to ensure accelerated ethics review in emergency situations, without undermining any of the substantive protections that ethics review is designed to provide. One option is to authorize the advance review of generic protocols for conducting research in outbreak conditions, which can then be rapidly adapted and reviewed for particular contexts. Early discussion and collaboration with local research ethics committees can help ensure the project is viable and can facilitate local committees' effective and efficient consideration of final protocols when an outbreak actually occurs.

- *Integrating research into broader outbreak response efforts* — National authorities and international organizations should seek to coordinate research projects in order to set priorities that are consistent with broader outbreak response efforts, and to avoid unnecessary duplication of research effort or competition among different sites. Researchers have an obligation to share information collected as part of a study if it is important for the ongoing response efforts, such as information about hidden cases and transmission chains or resistance to response measures. Persons who share the information and those who receive it should protect the confidentiality of personal information to the maximum extent possible. As part of the informed consent process, researchers should inform potential participants about the circumstances under which their personal information might be shared with public health authorities.

- *Ensuring that research does not drain critical health-related resources* — Research should not be done if it will excessively take away resources, including personnel, equipment, and health-care facilities, from other critical clinical and public health efforts. To the extent possible, research protocols should anticipate provisions for local capacity-building such as involving and training local contributors or, where possible, leaving behind any potentially useful tools or resources.

- *Confronting fear and desperation* — The climate of fear and desperation typical of infectious disease outbreaks can make it difficult for ethics committees or prospective participants to engage in an objective assessment of the risks and benefits of research participation. In an environment where large numbers of individuals become sick and die, any potential intervention may be perceived to be better than nothing, regardless of the risks and potential benefits actually involved. Those responsible for approving research protocols should ensure that clinical trials are not initiated unless there is a reasonable scientific basis to believe that the experimental intervention is likely to be safe and efficacious, and that the risks have been minimized to the extent reasonably possible. In addition, researchers and ethics committees should recognize that, during an outbreak, prospective participants may be especially prone to the therapeutic misconception — that is, the mistaken view that the intervention is primarily designed to directly benefit the individual participants, as opposed to developing generalizable knowledge for the potential benefit of persons in the future. Indeed, researchers themselves, as well as humanitarian aid workers, may some-times fail to distinguish between engaging in research and providing ordinary clinical care. Efforts should be made to dispel the therapeutic misconception to the extent reasonably possible. Despite such efforts, some prospective participants may still not fully appreciate the difference between research and ordinary medical care, and this should not in itself preclude their enrolment.

- *Addressing other barriers to informed consent* — In addition to the impact of fear and desperation, other factors can challenge researchers' ability to obtain informed consent to research; these range from cultural and linguistic differences between foreign researchers and local participants, to the fact that prospective participants in quarantine or isolation may be cut off from their families and other support systems and feel powerless to decline an invitation to participate in research. To the extent possible, consent processes compatible with international research ethics guidelines should be developed in consultation with local communities and implemented by locally recruited personnel. In addition, researchers should be well informed about the medical, psychological and social support systems available locally so that they can guide participants in need towards these services. In some situations, it may be necessary to develop rapid mechanisms for appointing proxy decision-makers, such as during outbreaks of diseases that affect cognitive abilities, or when an outbreak leaves a large number of children as orphans.

- ***Gaining and maintaining trust*** — Failure to build and maintain community trust during the process of research design and implementation, or when disclosing preliminary results, will not only impede study recruitment and completion but may also undermine the uptake of any interventions proven to be efficacious. Engaging with affected communities before, during, and after a study is essential to build and maintain trust. In environments in which the public's trust in government is fragile, researchers should remain as independent as possible from official public health activities. If government workers are themselves involved in conducting research, they should inform participants of this fact. Individuals who observe unethical practices carried out in the name of public health or emergency response efforts should promptly report them to ethics committees or other independent bodies.

- ***Selecting an appropriate research methodology*** — Exposing research participants to risk is ethically unacceptable if the study is not designed in a manner capable of providing valid results. It is therefore imperative that all research be designed and conducted in a methodologically rigorous manner. In clinical trials, the appropriateness of features such as randomization, placebo controls, blinding or masking should be determined on a case-by-case basis, with attention to both the scientific validity of the data and the acceptability of the methodology to the community from which participants will be drawn. In studies relying on qualitative methods, the potential benefits of using methodologies such as focus groups (in which individual confidentiality cannot be guaranteed) or of interviewing traumatized victims should be balanced against the risks and burdens to the individuals involved.

- ***Rapid data sharing***: As WHO has previously recognized, every researcher who engages in generation of information related to a public health emergency or acute public health event with the potential to progress to an emergency has the fundamental moral obligation to share preliminary results once they are adequately quality controlled for release.[16] Such information should be shared with public health officials, the study participants and affected population, and groups involved in wider international response efforts, without waiting for publication in scientific journals. Journals should facilitate this process by allowing researchers to rapidly disseminate information with immediate implications for public health without losing the opportunity for subsequent consideration for publication in a journal.[17]

- ***Assuring equitable access to the benefits of research*** — As recognized in existing international ethics guidelines, individuals and communities that participate in research should, where relevant, have access to any benefits that result from their participation. Research sponsors and host countries should agree in advance on mechanisms to ensure that any interventions found to be safe and effective in research will be made available to the local population without undue delay, including, when feasible, on a compassionate use basis before regulatory approval is finalized.

9. Emergency use of unproven interventions outside of research

> **Questions addressed:**
> • Under what circumstances is it ethically appropriate to offer patients unproven interventions outside clinical trials during infectious disease outbreaks?
> • How should such interventions be identified?
> • What type of ethical oversight should be conducted when unproven interventions are offered outside clinical trials during infectious disease outbreaks?
> • If such interventions are provided, what should individuals be told about them?
> • What obligations do persons administering unproven interventions outside clinical trials have to communicate with the community?
> • What obligations do persons administering unproven interventions outside clinical trials have to share the results?

There are many pathogens for which no proven effective intervention exists. For some pathogens there may be interventions that have shown promising safety and efficacy in the laboratory and in relevant animal models but that have not yet been evaluated for safety and efficacy in humans. Under normal circumstances, such interventions undergo testing in clinical trials that are capable of generating reliable evidence about safety and efficacy. However, in the context of an outbreak characterized by high mortality, it can be ethically appropriate to offer individual patients experimental interventions on an emergency basis outside clinical trials, provided:

1) no proven effective treatment exists;

2) it is not possible to initiate clinical studies immediately;

3) data providing preliminary support of the intervention's efficacy and safety are available, at least from laboratory or animal studies, and use of the intervention outside clinical trials has been suggested by an appropriately qualified scientific advisory committee on the basis of a favourable risk–benefit analysis;

4) the relevant country authorities, as well as an appropriately qualified ethics committee, have approved

such use;

    5) adequate resources are available to ensure that risks can be minimized;

    6) the patient's informed consent is obtained; and

    7) the emergency use of the intervention is monitored and the results are documented and shared in a timely manner with the wider medical and scientific community

As explained in prior WHO guidance, the use of experimental interventions under these circumstances is referred to as "monitored emergency use of unregistered and experimental interventions" (MEURI).[18]

Ethical basis for MEURI — MEURI is justified by the ethical principle of respect for patient autonomy — i.e. the right of individuals to make their own risk–benefit assessments in light of their personal values, goals and health conditions. It is also supported by the principle of beneficence — providing patients with available and reasonable opportunities to improve their condition, including measures that can plausibly mitigate extreme suffering and enhance survival.

Scientific basis for MEURI — Countries should not authorize MEURI unless it has first been recommended by an appropriately qualified scientific advisory committee especially established for this purpose. This committee should base its recommendations on a rigorous review of all data available from laboratory, animal and human studies of the intervention to assess the risk–benefit of MEURI in the context of the risks for patients who do not receive MEURI.

MEURI should be guided by the same ethical principles that guide use of unproven compounds in clinical trials, including the following:

- *Importance of ethical oversight* — MEURI is intended to be an exceptional measure for situations in which initiating a clinical trial is not feasible, not as a means to circumvent ethical oversight of the use of unproven interventions. Thus, mechanisms should be established to ensure that MEURI is subject to ethical oversight.

- *Effective resource allocation* — MEURI should not preclude or delay the initiation of clinical research into experimental products. In addition, it should not divert attention or resources from the implementation of effective clinical care and/or public health measures that may be crucial to control an outbreak.

- *Minimizing risk* — Administering unproven interventions necessarily involves risks, some of which will not be fully understood until further testing is conducted. However, any known risks associated with an intervention should be minimized to the extent reasonably possible (e.g. administration under hygienic conditions; using the same safety precautions that would be used during a clinical trial, with close monitoring and access to emergency medication and equipment; and providing necessary supportive treatment). Only investigational products manufactured according to good manufacturing practices should be used for MEURI.

- *Collection and sharing of meaningful data* — Physicians overseeing MEURI have the same moral obligation to collect all scientifically relevant data on the safety and efficacy of the intervention as researchers overseeing a clinical trial. Knowledge generated through MEURI should be aggregated across patients if possible and shared transparently, completely and rapidly with the MEURI scientific advisory committee, public health authorities, physicians and researchers in the country, and the international medical and scientific community. Information should be described accurately, without overstating benefits or understating uncertainties or risks

• *Importance of informed consent* — Individuals who are offered MEURI should be made aware that the intervention might not benefit them and might even harm them. The process of obtaining informed consent to MEURI should be carried out in a culturally and linguistically sensitive manner, with an emphasis on the content and understandability of the information conveyed and the voluntariness of the patient's decision. The ultimate choice of whether to receive the unproven intervention must rest with the patient, if the patient is in a condition to make the choice. If the patient is unconscious, cognitively impaired, or too sick to understand the information, proxy consent should be obtained from a family member or other authorized decision-maker.

• *Need for community engagement* — MEURI must be sensitive to local norms and practices. One way to try to ensure such sensitivity is to use rapid "community engagement teams" to promote dialogue about the potential benefits and risks of receiving interventions that have not yet been tested in clinical trials.

• *Fair distribution in the face of scarcity* — Compounds qualifying for MEURI may not be available in large quantities. In this situation, choices will have to be made about who receives each intervention. Countries should establish mechanisms for making these allocation decisions, taking into account the assessment of the MEURI Scientific Advisory Committee and the principles discussed in Guideline 4.

10. Rapid data sharing

> **Questions addressed:**
> • Why is rapid data sharing essential during an infectious disease outbreak?
> • What are the key ethical issues related to rapid data sharing?

The collection and sharing of data are essential parts of ordinary public health practice. During an infectious disease outbreak, data sharing takes on increased urgency because of the uncertain and ever-changing scientific information; the compromised response capacity of local health systems; and the heightened role of cross-border collaboration. For these reasons, "rapid data sharing is critical during an unfolding health emergency."[19] The ethically appropriate and rapid sharing of data can help identify etiological factors, predict disease spread, evaluate existing and novel treatment, symptomatic care and preventive measures, and guide the deployment of limited resources.

Activities that generate data include public health surveillance, clinical research studies, individual patient encounters (including MEURI), and epidemiological, qualitative, and environmental studies. All individuals and entities involved in these efforts should cooperate by sharing relevant and accurate data in a timely manner. As discussed in Guideline 8, efforts should be made to ensure that rapid sharing of information with immediate implications for public health does not preclude subsequent publication in a scientific journal.

As part of ongoing pre-epidemic preparedness efforts, countries should review their laws, policies, and practices regarding data sharing to ensure that they adequately protect the confidentiality of personal information and address other relevant ethical questions like managing incidental findings, and dealing with disputes over the ownership or control of information.

11. Long-term storage of biological specimens collected during infectious disease outbreaks

Questions addressed:

- What are the benefits and risks associated with the long-term storage of biological specimens collected during infectious disease outbreaks?
- What obligations do entities involved in the long-term storage of biological specimens collected during infectious disease outbreaks have to consult with the community?
- Are there any circumstances under which individuals should be asked for consent to, or given the opportunity to opt out of, the long-term storage of biological specimens collected during an infectious disease outbreak?
- What considerations should be taken into account in transferring biospecimens outside the institutions that collected them, whether domestically or internationally?

Biological specimens are often collected during an infectious disease outbreak in the context of diagnosis (e.g. to determine who has been infected with or exposed to a novel pathogen), surveillance (e.g. to identify the incidence of drug-resistant bacteria), or research (e.g. during clinical trials of new diagnostics, vaccines or interventions). Such samples are sent to laboratories on site or other laboratories, either domestically or internationally, for analysis.

Biospecimens collected during the management of an infectious disease outbreak offer researchers important opportunities to understand the outbreak pathogen better and to develop diagnostic, therapeutic, and preventive measures that may mitigate the harm of similar outbreaks in the future. At the same time, long-term storage of biospecimens involves potential risks to individuals and communities. Risks to individuals primarily relate to the unwanted disclosure of personal information. This can be minimized by protecting the confidentiality of individuals' identities, but confidentiality may be difficult to protect when only a small number of people are being tested. Moreover, even when individual confidentiality can be adequately protected, some individuals or communities might still be uncomfortable making their biospecimens available for future use, especially if such use is not subject to community control. Particular concerns can arise when specimens are transferred abroad without the originating country's prior agreement. Addressing these concerns requires time-consuming but necessary relationship-building, consultation, and education, as well as the establishment of policies, practices, and institutions capable of commanding public confidence and trust.

In addition to the general principles discussed elsewhere in this document, specific considerations relevant to the long-term storage of biological specimens collected during infectious disease outbreaks include the following:

- *Provision of information* — Before individuals are asked to provide biospecimens during an infectious disease outbreak, they should be given access to information about the purpose of the collection, whether their samples will be stored and, if so, the ways in which their specimens might be used in the future. When feasible and consistent with public health objectives, individuals should be asked to provide informed consent or be given the opportunity to opt out of the long-term storage of their specimens. Seeking informed consent is particularly important if there is any possibility that the specimens may later be used for research purposes

- *Community engagement* — Individuals and organizations involved in the long-term storage of biospecimens collected during infectious disease outbreaks should engage representatives of the local community in a dialogue about the process. Community representatives should be involved in the development of policies regarding future use of the samples, including measures to ensure that equitable access is provided to any benefits that result from using the samples in research.

- *International sharing of biospecimens* — Sharing biospecimens internationally may sometimes be necessary to conduct critical research. If it is necessary to transfer specimens internationally, appropriate governance mechanisms and regulatory systems should be established to ensure that representatives of the country where the specimens were collected are involved in decisions about the specimens' use. The international community should make efforts to strengthen countries' capacity to maintain biospecimens within their own borders.

- *Material transfer agreements* — Biospecimens should not be transferred outside of the countries from which they are collected without formal material transfer agreements. Such agreements should specify the purpose of the transfer, certify the specimen donor's consent as appropriate, provide for adequate confidentiality protection, cover the physical security of the specimens, require that the country of origin is acknowledged in future research reporting, and guarantee that the benefits of any subsequent use of the specimens will be shared with the communities from which the samples were obtained. Material transfer agreements should be developed with the involvement of persons responsible for the care of patients and the taking of samples, representatives of affected communities and patients, and relevant government officials and ethics committees.

12. Addressing sex- and gender-based differences

> **Questions addressed:**
>
> • How are sex and gender relevant to infectious disease outbreaks?
>
> • How can sex and gender be incorporated into public health and surveillance?
>
> • How can social and cultural practices relevant to gender roles affect infectious disease outbreaks?
>
> • How should appropriate reproductive health-care services be safely provided during an infectious disease outbreak?
>
> • How are sex and gender relevant to communication strategies during outbreaks?

Sex (biological and physiological characteristics) and gender (socially constructed roles, behaviours, activities, and attributes)[20] can influence the spread, containment, course, and consequences of infectious disease outbreaks. Sex and gender differences have been associated with differences in susceptibility to infection, levels of health care received, and in the course and outcome of illness.[21] Addressing sex and gender differences in infectious disease outbreak planning and response efforts requires attention to the following considerations:

• *Sex- and gender-inclusive surveillance programmes* — Public health surveillance should systematically collect disaggregated information on sex, gender, and pregnancy status, both to identify differential risks and modes of transmission, and to monitor any differential impact of an infectious disease outbreak and the interventions used to control it. This information is particularly important for pregnant women and their offspring.

• *Ensuring the availability of high-quality reproductive health-care services* — Whether or not they are currently pregnant, women of childbearing age should have access to the full range of high-quality reproductive health-care services during an infectious disease outbreak. These services should be organized and delivered in a manner that does not stigmatize persons who use them or expose them to a heightened risk of infection with the outbreak pathogen. If there is evidence that an infectious disease creates special risks for pregnant women or their fetus, both men and women should be informed of these risks and have access to safe methods to minimize them, along with reproductive counselling services.

- *Sex- and gender-inclusive research strategies* — Researchers should make efforts to ensure that studies do not disproportionately favour a particular sex or gender, and that women who are or might become pregnant are not inappropriately excluded from research participation. During an outbreak, research on experimental treatments and preventive measures should seek to identify any sex- or gender-related differences in outcomes.

- *Attention to social and cultural practices* — Gender-related roles and practices can affect all aspects of infectious disease outbreaks, including individuals' risk of becoming infected, the consequences of infection, their use of health services and other health-seeking behaviours, and their vulnerability to interpersonal violence. Policy-makers and outbreak responders should identify and respond to these factors, drawing when possible on relevant anthropological and sociological research.

- *Sex- and gender-sensitive communication strategies* — Entities responsible for developing and implementing communication strategies should be sensitive to sex- and gender-based differences in how individuals have access to and respond to health-related information. Separate messages and communication strategies may be needed to provide relevant information to particular subgroups, such as pregnant women or nursing mothers.

13. Frontline response workers' rights and obligations

Questions addressed:
- What obligations exist to protect the health of frontline workers who participate in infectious disease outbreak response efforts?
- What obligations exist to provide material support to frontline workers who participate in infectious disease outbreak response efforts?
- To what extent do these obligations extend to the workers' family?
- What should be taken into account in determining whether individuals have an obligation to serve as frontline workers during infectious disease outbreaks?
- What special obligations do workers in the health-care sector have during infectious disease outbreaks?

An effective infectious disease outbreak response depends on the contribution of a diverse range of frontline workers, some of whom may be working on a volunteer basis. These workers often assume considerable personal risk to carry out their jobs. Within the health-care sector, frontline workers range from health-care professionals with direct patient care responsibilities to traditional healers, ambulance drivers, laboratory workers, and hospital ancillary staff. Outside the health sector, individuals such as sanitation workers, burial teams, domestic humanitarian aid workers, and persons who carry out contact-tracing also play critical roles. Some of these workers may be among the least advantaged members of society, and have little control over the type of duties they are asked to perform. It is essential that frontline workers' rights and obligations be clearly established during the pre-outbreak planning period, in order to ensure that all actors are aware of what can reasonably be expected if an outbreak occurs.

Workers with certain professional qualifications, such as physicians, nurses, and funeral directors, may have a duty to assume a certain level of personal risk as part of their professional or employment commitments. Many frontline workers are not subject to any such obligations, and their assumption of risk must therefore be regarded as beyond the call of duty (i.e. "supererogatory"). This is particularly true for sanitation workers, burial teams, and community health workers, many of whom may have precarious employment contracts with no social protection, or work on a volunteer basis.

Regardless of whether a particular individual has a pre-existing duty to assume heightened risks during an infectious disease outbreak, once a worker has taken on these risks, society has a reciprocal obligation to provide necessary support. At a minimum, fulfilment of society's reciprocal obligations to frontline workers requires the following actions:

- *Minimizing the risk of infection* — Individuals should not be expected to take on risky work assignments during an infectious disease outbreak unless they are provided with the training, tools, and resources necessary to minimize the risks to the extent reasonably possible. This includes complete and accurate information known about the nature of the pathogen and infection control measures, updated information on the epidemiological situation at the local level, and the provision of personal protective equipment. Regular screening of frontline workers should be put in place to detect any infection as quickly as possible, in order to initiate immediate care and minimize the risk of transmission to colleagues, patients, families, and community members.

- *Priority access to health care* — Frontline workers who become sick, as well as any immediate family members who become ill through contact with the worker, should be ensured access to the highest level of care reasonably available. In addition, countries should consider giving frontline workers and their families priority access to vaccines and other treatments as they become available.

- *Appropriate remuneration* — Frontline workers should be given fair remuneration for their work. Governments should ensure that public sector workers are paid in a timely manner, and make efforts to ensure that actors in the private and nongovernmental sectors fulfil their own obligations to pay their employees and contractors. Fair remuneration for frontline workers includes the provision of financial support during periods in which workers are unable to carry out their normal responsibilities because of an infection acquired on the job.

- *Support for reintegrating into the community* — Frontline workers may experience stigma and discrimination, particularly those involved in unpopular measures such as infection control or burials not conducted according to the traditional customs. Governments should make efforts to reduce the risk of stigmatization and discrimination and help such workers to reintegrate into the community, including by providing job placement assistance and relocation to other communities if needed.

- *Assistance to family members* — Assistance should be provided to families of frontline workers who need to remain away from home in order to carry out their responsibilities or to recuperate from illness. Death benefits should be provided to family members of frontline workers who die in the line of duty, including those who were volunteers or "casual workers."

As noted above, some workers may have a duty to work during an infectious disease outbreak. However, even for these individuals, the duty to assume risk is not unlimited. In determining the scope of workers' duties to assume personal risks, the following factors should be taken into account:

- *Reciprocal obligations* — Any professional or employment-based obligation to assume personal risk is contingent on society's fulfilment of its reciprocal obligations to workers, as outlined above. If the reciprocal obligations are not met, frontline workers cannot legitimately be expected to assume a significant risk of harm to themselves and their families.

- *Risks and benefits* — Frontline workers should not be expected to expose themselves to risks that are disproportionate to the public health benefits their efforts are likely to achieve.

- *Equity and transparency* — Entities responsible for assigning frontline workers to specific tasks should ensure that risks are distributed among individuals and occupational categories in an equitable manner, and that the process of assigning workers is as transparent as possible.

- *Consequences for non-participation* — Frontline workers should be informed of the risks they are being asked to assume. Insofar as possible, expectations should be made clear in written employment agreements. Workers who are unwilling to accept reasonable risks and work assignments may be subject to professional repercussions (for example, loss of their job), but additional punishments, such as fines or imprisonment, are generally unwarranted. Persons responsible for assessing the consequences for non-participation should recognize that workers may sometimes need to balance other obligations, such as duty to family, against job-related responsibilities.

Additional obligations of those working in the health-care sector:

In addition to the issues addressed above, persons working in the health-care sector have obligations to the community during an infectious disease outbreak, including the following:

- *Participate in public health surveillance and reporting efforts* — Persons working in the health sector have an obligation to participate in organized measures to respond to infectious disease outbreaks, including public health surveillance and reporting. Health-care providers should protect the confidentiality of patient information to the maximum extent compatible with legitimate public health interests.

- *Provide accurate information to the public* — During an infectious disease outbreak, public health officials have the primary responsibility to communicate information about the outbreak pathogen, including how it is transmitted, how infection can be prevented, and what treatments or preventive measures may be effective. Those responsible for designing communication strategies should anticipate and respond to misinformation, exaggeration, and mistrust, and should seek (without withholding key information) to minimize the risk that information about risk factors will lead to stigmatization and discrimination. If persons working in the health sector are asked medical questions about the outbreak by patients or the general public, they should not spread unsubstantiated rumours or suspicion and ensure that information they provide comes from reliable sources.

- *Avoiding exploitation* — In the context of a rapidly spreading life-threatening illness with no proven treatment, desperate individuals may be willing to try any intervention offered, regardless of the expected risks or benefits. Health-care workers have a duty not to exploit individuals' vulnerability by offering treatments or preventive measures for which there is no reasonable basis to believe that the potential benefits outweigh the uncertainties and risks. This duty does not preclude the appropriate use of unproven interventions on an experimental basis, consistent with the guidelines set forth in Guideline 9.

14. Ethical issues in deploying foreign humanitarian aid workers

> **Questions addressed:**
>
> • What ethical issues arise in assigning foreign workers for deployment during infectious disease outbreaks?
>
> • What obligations do sponsoring organizations have to prepare foreign aid workers adequately for their missions?
>
> • What obligations do sponsoring organizations have regarding the conditions of deployment?
>
> • What obligations do sponsoring organizations have to coordinate with local officials?
>
> • What obligations do foreign aid workers have before, during, and after deployment?

Foreign governments and humanitarian aid organizations that deploy workers in infectious disease outbreaks have ethical obligations to both the workers themselves and the affected communities. These obligations include the following:

• *Coordination with local officials* — Foreign governments and external humanitarian aid organizations should deploy workers following discussion and agreement with local officials about their roles and responsibilities or, if this is not possible, with international organizations like WHO. Organizations working in a particular area should register their presence as a foreign Emergency Medical Team (EMT) with the local government, and have ongoing discussions among themselves and with the local government to clarify and coordinate their roles and responsibilities and address any disparities in standards of practice. Efforts should be coordinated with local authorities and care providers to ensure that the foreign agency does not excessively draw resources away from other essential services.

• *Fairness in assigning foreign workers for deployment* — Foreign aid workers should be deployed only if they are capable of providing necessary services not sufficiently available in the local setting. Assignment of foreign health workers should take into consideration their relevant skills and knowledge, as well as their linguistic and cultural competencies to meet mission objectives and understand and communicate with affected communities. It is inappropriate to deploy unqualified or unnecessary workers solely to satisfy their personal or professional desire to be helpful (so-called "disaster tourism").

• *Clarity about conditions of deployment* — Prospective foreign aid workers should be given comprehensive information about the project's expectations and risks so they can make informed decisions about whether or not they will be able to make appropriate contributions. In addition, foreign aid workers should be clearly informed of the conditions of their deployment, including the level of health care they can expect if they become ill, the circumstances under which they will be repatriated, available insurance, and whether benefits will be provided to their families in case of illness or death.

• *Provision of necessary training and resources* — Aid workers must be provided with appropriate training, preparation, and equipment to ensure that they can effectively carry out their mission with the lowest risks practicable. Training should include preparation in psychosocial and communication skills, and in understanding and respecting the local culture and traditions. Managers and organizations have an obligation to provide adequate support and guidance to the staff, both during their activity in the field and following their mission. This should include training and resources for managing challenging ethical issues, such as resource allocation decisions, triage, and inequities.

• *Ensuring the security and safety of aid workers* — Organizations that deploy foreign aid workers have an obligation to take all necessary measures to ensure the workers' security, particularly in situations of crisis; this obligation includes the provision of measures to reduce risks of exposure to infectious agents, contamination and violence. A clear chain of authority must be in place to provide oversight and ongoing advice. Individuals who object to assigned duties should have an opportunity for review and appeal, according to the norms of the organizations for which they work. Aid workers also have their own ethical obligations to patients, affected communities, their sponsoring organizations, and themselves. In addition to the obligations described in other sections of this document, obligations of foreign aid workers include the following:

• *Adequate preparation* — Aid workers should take part in any training that is offered. If they believe that the training they have been given is inadequate, they should bring their concerns to the attention of their organization managers. Foreign aid workers deployed during crises and where resources are scarce should carefully consider whether they are prepared to deal with ethical issues that may lead to moral and psychological distress.

• *Adherence to assigned roles and responsibilities* — Aid workers should understand the roles and responsibilities they have been asked to assume and should not, except in the most extreme circumstances, undertake tasks they have not been authorized to perform. In addition, they should provide clear and timely information to both their sponsoring organizations and local officials and should understand that, if they go beyond the tasks they have been authorized to perform, they will be accountable not only within their own organizations but also under applicable local standards and laws.

- ***Attention to appropriate infection control practices*** — Aid workers should be vigilant in adhering to infection control practices, both for their own protection and to prevent further transmission of disease. Aid workers should follow recommended protocols for monitoring symptoms and reporting their health status (including possible pregnancy), before, during and after their service.

References

1 Resolution WHA58.3. Revision of the International Health Regulations. In: Fifty-eighth World Health Assembly, Geneva, 16–25 May 2005. Resolutions and decisions, annex. Geneva: World Health Organization; 2005 (WHA58/2005/REC/1; http://apps.who.int/gb/ebwha/pdf_files/WHA58-REC1/english/A58_2005_REC1-en.pdf, accessed 23 July 2016) .

2 Addressing ethical issues in pandemic influenza planning: Discussion papers. Geneva: World Health Organization; 2008 (WHO/HSE/EPR/GIP/2008.2, WHO/IER/ETH/2008.1; http://apps.who.int/iris/bitstream/10665/69902/1/WHO_IER_ETH_2008.1_eng.pdf?ua=1, accessed 23 July 2016) .

3 Guidance on ethics of tuberculosis prevention, care and control. Geneva: World Health Organization; 2010 (WHO/HTM/TB/2010.16, http://apps.who.int/iris/bitstream/10665/44452/1/9789241500531_eng.pdf?ua=1, accessed 23 July 2016) .

4 Ethics of using convalescent whole blood and convalescent plasma during the Ebola epidemic. Geneva: World Health Organization; 2015 (WHO/HIS/KER/GHE/15.1; http://apps.who.int/iris/bitstream/10665/161912/1/WHO_HIS_KER_GHE_15.1_eng .pdf?ua=1&ua=1, accessed 23 July 2016) .

5 Ethical considerations for use of unregistered interventions for Ebola viral disease. Geneva: World Health Organization; 2014 (WHO/HIS/KER/GHE/14.1, http://apps.who.int/iris/bitstream/10665/130997/1/WHO_HIS_KER_GHE_14.1_eng.pdf?ua=1, accessed 23 July 2016) .

6 Becker L. Reciprocity, justice, and disability. Ethics. 2005;116(1):9–39 .

7 Dawson A, Jennings B. The place of solidarity in public health ethics. Public Health Reviews. 2012;34(1):65–79 .

8 Siracusa Principles on the Limitation and Derogation Provision in the International Covenant on Civil and Political Rights. Geneva: American Association for the International Commission of Jurists; 1985 (http://icj.wpengine.netdna-cdn.com/wp-content/uploads/1984/07/Siracusa-principles-ICCPR-legal-submission-1985-eng.pdf, accessed 23 July 2016) .

9 United Nations Economic and Social Council. General Comment No. 14: The right to Highest Attainable Standard of Health (Art. 12 of the International Covenant on Economic, Social and Cultural Rights). New York: United Nations Committee on Economic, Social and Cultural Rights (E/C. 12/2000/4 – 2000; www1.umn.edu/humanrts/gencomm/escgencom14.htm, accessed 23 July 2016) .

10 Parpia AS, Ndeffo-Mbah ML, Wenzel NS, Galvani AP. Effects of response to the 2014–2015 Ebola outbreak on deaths from malaria, HIV/AIDS, and tuberculosis, West Africa. Emerg Infect Dis. 2016;22(3)

(http://dx.doi.org/10.3201/eid2203.150977, accessed 23 July 2016) .

11 Declaration of Helsinki – Ethical principles for medical research involving human subjects, revised October 2013 Ferney-Voltaire: World Medical Association; 2013 (www.wma.net/en/30publications/10policies/b3/index.html, accessed 23 July 2016) .

12 International ethical guidelines for biomedical research involving human subjects. Geneva: Council for International Organizations of Medical Sciences; 2002 (www.cioms.ch/publications/guidelines/guidelines_nov_2002_blurb.htm, accessed 23 July 2016) .

13 Standards and operational guidance for ethics review of health-related research with human participants. Geneva: World Health Organization; 2011 (www.who.int/ethics/publications/9789241502948/en/, accessed 23 July 2016) .

14 Ethics in epidemics, emergencies and disasters: Research, surveillance and patient care. Geneva: World Health Organization; 2015 (who.int/ethics/publications/epidemics-emergencies-research/en/, accessed 23 July 2016) .

15 Research ethics in international epidemic response. Geneva: World Health Organization; 2009 (WHO/HSE/GIP/ITP/10.1; www.who.int/ethics/gip_research_ethics_.pdf, accessed 23 July 2016) .

16 Developing global norms for sharing data and results during public health emergencies. Geneva: World Health Organization; 2015 (www.who.int/medicines/ebola-treatment/blueprint_phe_data-share-results/en/, accessed 23 July 2016) .

17 Overlapping publications. International Committee of Medical Journal Editors (www.icmje.org/recommendations/browse/publishing-and-editorial-issues/overlapping-publications.html, accessed 23 July 2016) .

18 Ethical issues related to study design for trials on therapeutics for Ebola Virus Disease.2014. Report of the WHO Ethics Working Group meeting, 20–21 October 2014. Geneva: World Health Organization; 2014 (WHO/HIS/KER/GHE/14.2; http://apps.who.int/iris/bitstream/10665/137509/1/WHO_HIS_KER_GHE_14.2_eng.pdf, accessed 23 July 2016) .

19 Dye C, Bartolomeos K, Moorthy V, Kieny MP. Data sharing in public health emergencies: a call to researchers. Bull World Health Organ. 2016;1:94(3):158. doi: 10.2471/BLT.16.170860 (www.who.int/bulletin/volumes/94/3/16-170860.pdf?ua=1) .

20 Gender, women and health. In: WHO [website]. Geneva: World Health Organization (http://apps.who.int/gender/whatisgender/en/, accessed 23 July 2016) .

21 Addressing sex and gender in epidemic-prone infectious diseases. Geneva: World Health Organization; 2007 (www.who.int/csr/resources/publications/SexGenderInfectDis.pdf) .

Annex 1. Ethics guidance documents that contributed to the *Guidance for managing ethical issues in infectious disease outbreaks*

WHO guidance documents

Addressing ethical issues in pandemic influenza planning: Discussion papers. Geneva: World Health Organization; 2008 (WHO/HSE/EPR/GIP/2008.2, WHO/IER/ETH/2008.1; http://apps.who.int/iris/bitstream/10665/69902/1/WHO_IER_ETH_2008.1_eng.pdf?ua=1) .

Ethical considerations for use of unregistered interventions for Ebola viral disease. Report of an advisory panel to WHO. Geneva: World Health Organization; 2014 (WHO/HIS/KER/ GHE/14.1; http://apps.who.int/iris/bitstream/10665/130997/1/WHO_HIS_KER_GHE_14.1_eng.pdf?ua=1) .

Ethical considerations in developing a public health response to pandemic influenza. Geneva: World Health Organization; 2007 (WHO/CDS/EPR/GIP/2007.2; http://www.who.int/csr/resources/publications/WHO_CDS_EPR_GIP_2007_2c.pdf?ua=1) .

Ethical issues related to study design for trials on therapeutics for Ebola virus disease. WHO Ethics Working Group Meeting, 20–21 October 2014. Geneva: World Health Organization; 2014 (WHO/HIS/KER/GHE/14.2; http://apps.who.int/iris/bitstream/10665/137509/1/WHO_HIS_KER_GHE_14.2_eng.pdf?ua=1) .

Ethics of using convalescent whole blood and convalescent plasma during the Ebola epidemic: Interim guidance for ethics review committees, researchers, national health authorities and blood transfusion services. Geneva: World Health Organization; 2015 (http://apps.who.int/iris/bitstream/10665/161912/1/WHO_HIS_KER_GHE_15.1_eng .pdf?ua=1&ua=1) .

Ethics in epidemics, emergencies and disasters: Research, surveillance and patient care: Training manual. Geneva: World Health Organization; 2015 (http://apps.who.int/iris/bitstream/10665/196326/1/9789241549349_eng.pdf?ua=1) .

Guidance on ethics of tuberculosis prevention, care and control. Geneva: World Health Organization; 2010 (http://apps.who.int/iris/bitstream/10665/44452/1/9789241500531_eng.pdf?ua=1) .

Research ethics in international epidemic response: WHO Technical Consultation. Geneva: World Health Organization; 2009 (www.who.int/ethics/gip_research_ethics_.pdf) .

Standards and operational guidance for ethics review of health-related research with hu-

man participants. Geneva: World Health Organization; 2011 (http://apps.who.int/iris/bitstre
am/10665/44783/1/9789241502948_eng.pdf?ua=1&ua=1) .

National guidance/opinion papers

Allocation of ventilators in an influenza pandemic: Planning document. New York State Task
Force on Life and the Law; 2007 (www.cidrap.umn.edu/sites/default/files/public/php/196/196_guid-
ance.pdf) .

Altevogt BM, Stroud C, Hanson S, Hanfling D, Gostin LO, editors. Guidance for establishing crisis standards of care for use in disaster situations: A letter report. Washington: National Academies
Press; 2009 (www.nap.edu/read/12749/chapter/1) .

Ethical issues raised by a possible influenza pandemic. Opinion No. 106. Paris: National Consultative Ethics Committee for Health and Life Sciences; 2009 (www.ccne-ethique.fr/sites/default/files/
publications/avis_106_anglais.pdf) .

Ethics and Ebola: Public health planning and response. Washington DC: Presidential Commission for the Study of Bioethical Issues.; 2015 (http://bioethics.gov/sites/default/files/Ethics-and-Ebo-
la_PCSBI_508.pdf) .

Ethical guidelines in Pandemic Influenza - Recommendations of the Ethics Subcommittee of
the Advisory Committee to the Director, United States Centers for Disease Control and Prevention.
Ethical guidelines in pandemic influenza. Atlanta: Centers for Disease Control and Prevention; 2007
(www.cdc.gov/od/science/integrity/phethics/docs/panflu_ethic_guidelines.pdf) .

Ethics Subcommittee of the Advisory Committee to the Director, United States Centers for Disease Control and Prevention. Ethical guidance for public health emergency preparedness and response: Highlighting ethics and values in vital public health service. Atlanta: Centers for Disease
Control and Prevention; 2008 (www.cdc.gov/od/science/integrity/phethics/docs/white_paper_final_
for_website_2012_4_6_12_final_for_web_508_compliant.pdf) .

Ethics Subcommittee of the Advisory Committee to the Director, United States Centers for Disease Control and Prevention. Ethical considerations for decision making regarding allocation of mechanical ventilators during a severe influenza pandemic or other public health emergency. Atlanta:
Centers for Disease Control and Prevention; 2011 (www.cdc.gov/about/pdf/advisory/ventdocument_
release.pdf) .

Integrated national avian and pandemic influenza response plan, 2007–2009. In: Avian Influenza
and the Pandemic Threats: Nigeria. Geneva: United Nations System Influenza Coordination Office
(http://un-influenza.org/?q=content/Nigeria) .

National Advisory Board on Health Care Ethics. Ethical considerations related to preparedness for a pandemic. Helsinki: Ministry of Social Affairs and Health; 2005 (http://etene.fi/docu-

ments/1429646/1561478/2005+Statement+on+ethical+considerations+related+to+preparedness+-for+a+pandemic.pdf/fc3f2412-acfc-4685-b427-ca710a43c103) .

National Ethics Advisory Committee. Getting through together: Ethical values for a pandemic. Wellington: Ministry of Health; 2007 (https://neac.health.govt.nz/system/files/documents/publications/getting-through-together-jul07.pdf) .

Notes on the interim US guidance for monitoring and movement of persons with potential Ebola virus exposure. Atlanta GA: Centers for Disease Control and Prevention; 2016 (www .cdc.gov/vhf/ebola/exposure/monitoring-and-movement-of-persons-with-exposure.html) .

Pandemic Influenza Ethics Initiative Workgroup. Meeting the challenge of pandemic influenza: Ethical guidance for leaders and health care professionals in the veterans health administration. Washington DC: National Center for Ethics in Health Care, Veterans Health Administration; 2010 (www.ethics.va.gov/docs/pandemicflu/Meeting_the_Challenge_of_Pan_Flu-Ethical_Guidance_VHA_20100701.pdf) .

Responding to pandemic influenza: The ethical framework for policy and planning. London: Department of Health; 2007 (www.gov.scot/Resource/Doc/924/0054555.pdf) .

Stand on guard for thee: Ethical considerations in preparedness planning for pandemic influenza. Toronto: University of Toronto Joint Centre for Bioethics; 2005 (www.jcb.utoronto.ca/people/documents/upshur_stand_guard.pdf) .

Swiss Federal Office of Public Health. Swiss Influenza Pandemic Plan. Bern; 2013 (www.bag.admin.ch/influenza/01120/01132/10097/10104/index.html?lang=en&download=NHzLpZeg7t,lnp6I0NTU042l2Z6ln1ad1IZn4Z2qZpnO2Yuq2Z6gpJCGenx6gWym162epYbg2c_JjKbNoKSn6A--) .

Venkat A, Wolf L, Geiderman JM, Asher SL, Marco CA, McGreevy J et al. Ethical issues in the response to Ebola virus disease in US emergency departments: a position paper of the American College of Emergency Physicians, the Emergency Nurses Association and the Society for Academic Emergency Medicine. J Emerg Nurs. 2015; Mar;41(2):e5-e16. doi:10.1016/j.jen.2015.01.012 (www.ncbi.nlm.nih.gov/pubmed/25770003) .

Annex 2. Participants at meetings to formulate *Guidance for managing ethical issues in infectious disease outbreaks*

Panel discussion: Ethical considerations for use of unregistered interventions for Ebola viral disease, World Health Organization, Geneva, 11 August 2014

Advisors

Dr Juan Pablo Beca, Professor, Bioethics Center, Universidad del Desarrollo, Chile

Dr Helen Byomire Ndagije, Head, Drug Information Department, Ugandan National Drug Authority, Uganda

Dr Philippe Calain (Chair), Senior Researcher, Unit of Research on Humanitarian Stakes and Practices, Médecins Sans Frontières, Switzerland

Dr Marion Danis, Head, Ethics and Health Policy and Chief, Bioethics Consultation Service, National Institutes of Health, United States of America

Professor Jeremy Farrar, Director, Wellcome Trust, United Kingdom

Professor Ryuichi Ida, Chair, National Bioethics Advisory Committee, Japan

Professor Tariq Madani, infectious diseases physician and clinical academic researcher, Saudi Arabia

Professor Michael Selgelid, Director, Centre for Human Bioethics, Monash University, Australia

Professor Peter Smith, Professor of Tropical Epidemiology, London School of Tropical Medicine and Hygiene, United Kingdom

Ms Jeanine Thomas, Patient Safety Champion, United States of America

Professor Aisssatou Touré, Head, Immunology Department, Institut Pasteurde Dakar,,Senegal

Professor Ross Upshur, Chair in Primary Care Research; Professor, Department of Family and Community Medicine and Dalla Lana School of Public Health, University of Toronto; Canada

Resource persons

Dr Daniel Bausch, Head, Virology and Emerging Infections Department, US Naval Medical Research Unit No. 6, Peru

Professor Luciana Borio, Assistant Commissioner for Counterterrorism Policy; Director, Office of

Counterterrorism and Emerging Threats, Food and Drug Administration, United States of America

Dr Frederick Hayden, Professor of Clinical Virology and Professor of Medicine, University of Virginia School of Medicine, United States of America

Dr Stephan Monroe, Deputy Director, National Centre for Emerging and Zoonotic Infectious Diseases, Centers for Disease Control and Prevention, United States of America

WHO Secretariat

WHO headquarters, Geneva, Switzerland

Dr Margaret Chan, Director-General

Dr Marie-Paule Kieny, Assistant Director-General, Health Systems and Innovation

Dr Marie-Charlotte Bouesseau, Ethics Advisor, Service Delivery and Safety

Dr Pierre Formenty, Scientist, Control of Epidemic Diseases, Department of Pandemic and Epidemic Diseases

Dr Margaret Harris, Communication Officer, Department of Pandemic and Epidemic Diseases

Mr Gregory Hartl, Coordinator, Department of Communications

Dr Rüdiger Krech, Director, Health Systems and Innovation

Dr Andreas Reis, Technical Officer, Global Health Ethics, Department of Knowledge, Ethics and Research

Dr Cathy Roth, Adviser, Office of the Assistant Director-General, Health Systems and Innovation

Dr Vasee Sathyamoorthy, Technical Officer, Initiative for Vaccine Research, Department of Immunization, Vaccines and Biologicals

Dr Abha Saxena, Coordinator, Global Health Ethics, Department of Knowledge, Ethics and Research

Dr David Wood, Coordinator, Technologies Standards and Norms, Department of Essential Medicines and Health Products

Regional offices

Dr Marion Motari, Partnership and Resource Mobilization, Regional Office for Africa, Brazzaville, Congo

Dr Martin Ota, Medical Officer, Health Information and Knowledge Management, Regional Office for Africa, Brazzaville, Congo

Dr Carla Saenz, Bioethics Advisor, Regional Office for the Americas, Washington DC, United States of America

Consultation on potential Ebola therapies and vaccines: Pre-meeting of the Ethics Working Group, World Health Organization, Geneva, 3 September 2014

Participants

Professor Clement Adebamowo, Chair, National Research Ethics Committee, Nigeria

Dr Philippe Calain, Senior Researcher, Unit of Research on Humanitarian Stakes and Practices, Médecins Sans Frontières, Switzerland

Dr Marion Danis, Head, Ethics and Health Policy and Chief, Bioethics Consultation Service, National Institutes of Health, United States of America

Professor Jeremy Farrar, Director, Wellcome Trust, United Kingdom

Professor Jennifer Gibson, Sun Life Financial Chair in Bioethics; Director, Joint Centre for Bioethics; and Associate Professor, Institute of Health Policy, Management and Evaluation, University of Toronto, Canada

Ms Robinah Kaitiritimba, Patient Representative (community representative, Makerere University Institutional Review Boards; Uganda National Health Consumers' Organisation), Uganda

Dr Bocar Kouyate, Special Advisor to the Minister of Health (former Chair of National Ethics Committee), Burkina Faso

Professor Cheikh Niang, Université Cheikh Anta Diop, Senegal

Professor Michael Selgelid,Director, Centre for Human Bioethics, Monash University, Australia

Professor Oyewale Tomori (Chair), President, Nigeria National Academy of Sciences, Nigeria

Dr Aissatou Touré (Co-Chair), Head, Immunology Department, Institut Pasteur de Dakar and Member, National Ethics Committee, Senegal

WHO Secretariat

WHO headquarters, Geneva, Switzerland

Dr Andreas Reis, Technical Officer, Global Health Ethics, Department of Knowledge, Ethics and Research

Dr Abha Saxena, Coordinator, Global Health Ethics, Department of Knowledge, Ethics and Research

WHO Regional Office

Dr Carla Saenz, Bioethics Advisor, Regional Office for the Americas, Washington DC, United States of America

Ethical issues related to study design for trials on therapeutics, World Health Organization, Geneva, 20–21 October 2014

Ethics Working Group

Professor Arthur Caplan, Drs William F and Virginia Connolly Mitty; Director, Division of Medical Ethics, New York University Langone Medical Center's Department of Population Health, United States of America

Dr Clare Chandler, Senior Lecturer, Medical Anthropology, Department of Global Health and Development, London School of Hygiene and Tropical Medicine, United Kingdom

Dr Alpha Ahmadou Diallo, Administrator, National Ethics Committee, Ministry of Health and Public Hygiene, Guinea

Dr Amar Jesani, Independent Researcher and Teacher, Bioethics and Public Health; Editor, Indian Journal of Medical Ethics; Visiting Professor, Centre for Ethics, Yenepoya University, India

Dr Dan O'Connor, Head, Medical Humanities, Wellcome Trust, United Kingdom

Dr Lisa Schwartz, Arnold L. Johnson Chair in Health Care Ethics, McMaster Ethics in Healthcare, McMaster University, Canada

Professor Michael Selgelid, Director, Centre for Human Bioethics, Monash University, Australia

Dr Paulina Tindana, Ethicist and Senior Researcher, Navrongo Health Research Centre, Ghana

Professor Ross Upshur, Chair in Primary Care Research; Professor, Department of Family and Community Medicine and Dalla Lana School of Public Health, University of Toronto, Canada

Invited participants

Dr Enrica Alteri, Head, Human Medicines Evaluation Division, European Medicines Agency, United Kingdom

Dr Nicholas Andrews, Statistics Modelling and Economics Department, Centre for Infectious Disease Surveillance and Control, Public Health England, United Kingdom

Professor Oumou Younoussa Bah-Sow, Head of Pneumophtisiology, Ignace Deen National Hospital, Guinea

Dr Luciana Borio, Assistant Commissioner for Counterterrorism Policy; Director, Office of Counterterrorism and Emerging Threats, Food and Drug Administration, United States of Ameria

Dr Jacob Thorup Cohn; Vice President, Governmental Affairs, Bavarian Nordic, Denmark

Dr Edward Cox, Director, Office of Antimicrobial Products, Office of New Drugs Center for Drug Evaluation and Research, Food and Drug Administration, Silver Spring MD, United States of America

Dr Nicolas Day, Director, Thailand/Laos Wellcome Trust Major Overseas Programme Mahidol-Oxford Tropical Medicine Research Unit, Thailand

Dr Matthias Egger, Professor, Clinical Epidemiology, Department of Social Medicine, University of Bristol, United Kingdom; Epidemiology and Public Health, Institute for Social and Preventive Medicine, University of Bern, Switzerland

Dr Elizabeth Higgs, Global Health Science Advisor, Office of the Director, Division of Clinical Research, National Institute of Allergy and Infectious Diseases, National Institutes of Health, United States of America

Dr Nadia Khelef, Senior Advisor, Global Affairs, Institut Pasteur, France

Professor Trudie Lang, Lead Professor, Global Health Network, Nuffield Department of Medicine, University of Oxford, United Kingdom

Dr Matthew Lim, Senior Advisor, Global Health Security, Department of Health and Human Services, United States of America

Professor Ira Longini, Professor of Biostatistics, Department of Biostatistics, College of Public Health and College of Medicine, University of Florida, United States of America

Colonel Scott Miller, Director, Infectious Disease Clinical Research Program, Department of Preventive Medicine, Uniformed Services University, United States of America

Ms Adeline Osakwe, Head, National Pharmacovigilance Centre, National Agency for Food and Drug Administration and Control, Nigeria

Ms Virginie Pirard, Member, Belgian Advisory Committee on Bioethics; Ethics Advisor, Institut Pasteur, France

Dr Micaela Serafini, Medical Director, Médecins Sans Frontières, Switzerland

Mr Jemee Tegli, Institutional Review Board Administrator, University of Liberia–Pacific Institute for Research and Evaluation Institutional Review Board, Liberia

Dr Gervais Tougas, Representative, International Federation of Pharmaceutical Manufacturers & Associations, Chief Medical Officer, Novartis, Switzerland

Dr Johan van Griensven, Department of Clinical Sciences, Institute of Tropical Medicine, Belgium

Professor John Whitehead, Emeritus Professor, Department of Mathematics and Statistics, Fylde College, Lancaster University, United Kingdom

WHO Secretariat

Dr Marie-Paule Kieny, Assistant Director-General, Health Systems and Innovation

Dr Marie-Charlotte Bouesseau, Advisor, Department of Service Delivery and Safety

Dr Vania de la Fuente-Núñez, Technical Officer, Global Health Ethics, Department of Knowledge, Ethics and Research

Dr Martin Friede, Scientist, Public Health, Innovation and Intellectual Property, Department of Essential Medicines and Health Products

Ms Marisol Guraiib, Technical Officer, Global Health Ethics, Department of Knowledge, Ethics and Research

Ms Corinna Klingler, Intern, Global Health Ethics, Department of Knowledge, Ethics and Research

Dr Selena Knight, Intern, Global Health Ethics, Department of Knowledge, Ethics and Research

Dr Nicola Magrini, Scientist, Policy, Access and Use, Department of Essential Medicines and Health Products

Dr Cathy Roth, Adviser, Office of the Assistant Director-General, Health Systems and Innovation

Dr Vasee Sathiyamoorthy, Technical Officer, Initiative for Vaccine Research, Department of Immunization, Vaccines and Biologicals

Dr Abha Saxena, Coordinator, Global Health Ethics, Department of Knowledge, Ethics and Research

Dr David Wood, Coordinator, Technologies, Standards and Norms, Department of Essential Medicines and Health Products

Developing ethics guidelines for public health responses during epidemics, including for the conduct of related research, Dublin, Ireland, 25–26 May 2015

Participants

Dr Annick Antierens, Manager, Investigational Platform for Experimental Ebola Products, Médecins Sans Frontières, Switzerland

Dr Philippe Calain, Senior Researcher, Unit of Research on Humanitarian Stakes and Practices, Médecins Sans Frontières, Switzerland

Dr Edward Cox, Director, Office of Antimicrobial Products, Food and Drug Administration, United States of America

Professor Heather Draper, Professor of Biomedical Ethics, University of Birmingham, United Kingdom

Dr Sarah Edwards, Senior Lecturer in Research Ethics and Governance, University College London, United Kingdom

Professor Jónína Einarsdóttir, Medical Anthropology, School of Social Sciences, University of Iceland, Iceland

Professor Jeremy Farrar, Director, Wellcome Trust, United Kingdom

Dr Margaret Fitzgerald, Public Health Specialist, Irish Health Service Executive, Ireland

Dr Gabriel Fitzpatrick, Médecins Sans Frontières, Ireland

Ms Lorraine Gallagher, Development Specialist, Irish Aid, Department of Foreign Affairs, Ireland

Professor Jennifer Gibson, Sun Life Financial Chair in Bioethics; Director, Joint Centre for Bioethics; Associate Professor, Institute of Health Policy, Management and Evaluation, University of Toronto, Canada

Professor Frederick G Hayden, Professor of Medicine and Pathology, University of Virginia School of Medicine, Unites States of America

Dr Rita Helfand, Centers for Disease Control and Prevention, United States of America

Dr Simon Jenkins, Research Fellow, University of Birmingham Project on the ethical challenges experienced by British military healthcare professionals in the Ebola region, United Kingdom

Dr Pretesh Kiran, Assistant Professor, Community Health; Convener, Disaster Management Unit, St Johns National Academy of Health Sciences, India

Dr Markus Kirchner, Department for Infectious Disease Epidemiology, Robert Koch Institute, Germany

Dr Katherine Littler, Senior Policy Adviser, Wellcome Trust, United Kingdom

Professor Samuel McConkey, Head, International Health and Tropical Medicine, Royal College of Surgeons, Ireland

Dr Farhat Moazam, Founding Chairperson, Center of Biomedical Ethics and Culture, Sindh Institute of Urology and Transplantation, Pakistan

Dr Robert Nelson, Deputy Director and Senior Pediatric Ethicist, Office of Pediatric Therapeutics, Food and Drug Administration, United States of America

Professor Alistair Nichol, Consultant Anaesthetist, School of Medicine and Medical Sciences, and EU projects, University College Dublin, Ireland

Professor Lisa Schwartz, Arnold Johnson Chair in Health Care Ethics, Ethics in Health Care, McMaster University, Canada

Professor Michael Selgelid, Director, Centre for Human Bioethics, Monash University, Australia

Dr Kadri Simm, Associate Professor of Practical Philosophy, University of Tartu, Estonia

Dr Aissatou Touré, Head, Immunology Department, Institut Pasteur de Dakar and Member, National Ethics Committee, Senegal

Professor Ross Upshur, Canada Research Chair in Primary Care Research; Professor, Department of Family and Community Medicine and Dalla Lana School of Public Health, University of Toronto, Canada

Dr Maria Van Kerkhove, Centre for Global Health, Institut Pasteur, France

Dr Aminu Yakubu, Department of Health Planning and Research, Federal Ministry of Health, Nigeria

Resource person

Professor Carl Coleman (Rapporteur), Professor of Law and Academic Director, Division of On-line Learning, Seton Hall University, New Jersey, United States of America

WHO headquarters Secretariat, Geneva, Switzerland

Dr Vania de la Fuente-Núñez, Technical Officer, Global Health Ethics, Department of Knowledge, Ethics and Research

Dr Andreas Reis, Technical Officer, Global Health Ethics, Department of Knowledge, Ethics and Research

Dr Abha Saxena, Coordinator, Global Health Ethics, Department of Knowledge, Ethics and Research

Meeting to develop WHO Guidance on ethics and epidemics. Prato, Italy, 22–24 November 2015

Participants

Dr Franklyn Prieto Alvarado, Universidad Nacional de Colombia, Colombia

Dr Annick Antierens, Médecins Sans Frontières, Switzerland

Professor Oumou Younoussa Bah-Sow, Ignace Deen National Hospital, Guinea

Dr Ruchi Baxi, The Ethox Centre, United Kingdom

Dr Ron Bayer, Mailman School of Public Health, United States of America

Dr Oscar Cabrera, Executive Director, O'Neill Institute for National and Global Health Law, Georgetown University Law Center, United States of America

Dr Philippe Calain, Senior Researcher, Research on Humanitarian Stakes and Practices, Médecins Sans Frontières, Switzerland

Dr Voo Teck Chuan, National Academy of Health Sciences, India

Professor Alice Desclaux, Institut de Recherche pour le Développement, Unité TRANSVIHMI, Centre Régional de Recherche et de Formation sur le VIH et les Maladies Associées, Hôpital de Fann, Sénégal

Dr Benedict Dossen, National Research Ethics Board, University of Liberia–Pacific Institute for Research and Evaluation, Africa Center Institutional Review Board, Liberia

Dr Sarah Edwards, Research Ethics and Governance, University College London, United Kingdom

Professor Amy F Fairchild, Mailman School of Public Health, United States of America

Dr Eddy Foday, Ministry of Health and Sanitation, Sierra Leone

Professor Frederick G Hayden, Mailman School of Public Health, United States of America

Dr Amar Jesani, Yenepoya University, India

Ms Rebecca Johnson, Ebola survivor, Sierra Leone

Ms Robinah Kaitiritimba, Patient representative (Community representative, Makerere University Institutional Review Board; Uganda National Health Consumers' Organisation, Uganda

Dr Stephen Kennedy, Coordinator, Ebola Virus Disease Research, Incident Management System, Liberia

Dr Pretesh Kiran, National Academy of Health Sciences, India

Dr Bocar Kouyate, Special Advisor to the Minister of Health, Burkina Faso Professor Mark Leys, Vrije Universiteit Brussel, Belgium

Dr Farhat Moazam, Founding Chairperson of Center of Biomedical Ethics and Culture, Sindh Institute of Urology and Transplantation, Pakistan

Dr Dónal O'Mathúna, Dublin City University, Ireland

Professor Mahmudur Rahman, Director, Institute of Epidemiology, Disease Control and Research; National Influenza Center, Ministry of Health and Family Welfare, Bangladesh

Professor Lisa Schwartz, Arnold Johnson Chair in Health Care Ethics, McMaster Ethics in Healthcare, McMaster University, Canada

Professor Michael Selgelid, Director, Centre for Human Bioethics, Monash University, Australia Dr Aissatou Touré, Head, Immunology Unit, Institut Pasteur de Dakar, Senegal

Dr Maria Van Kerkhove, Centre for Global Health, Institut Pasteur, France

Observer

Dr Katherine Littler, Senior Policy Adviser, Policy Department, Wellcome Trust, United Kingdom

Resource consultants

Professor Carl Coleman, Professor of Law and Academic Director, Division of Online Learning, Seton Hall University, New Jersey, United States of America

Dr Michele Loi (Rapporteur), Post-doctoral research fellow, ETH Zürich, Switzerland

Dr Diego Silva, Assistant Professor, Faculty of Health Sciences, Simon Fraser University, Canada

WHO headquarters Secretariat, Geneva, Switzerland

Dr Pierre Formenty, Scientist, Control of Epidemic Diseases, Department of Pandemic and Epidemic Diseases

Dr Vania de la Fuente-Núñez,Technical Officer, Global Health Ethics, Department of Knowledge, Ethics and Research

Dr Andreas Reis, Technical Officer Global Health Ethics, Department of Knowledge, Ethics and Research

Dr Abha Saxena, Coordinator, Global Health Ethics, Department of Knowledge, Ethics and Research